T5-BAF-239

Am I Still a Woman?

Hysterectomy and Gender Identity

Am I Still a Woman?

Hysterectomy
and Gender Identity

Jean Elson

 Temple University Press
Philadelphia

WHITE PLAINS PUBLIC LIBRARY
WHITE PLAINS, NEW YORK 10601

Temple University Press, Philadelphia 19122
Copyright © 2004 by Temple University
All rights reserved
Published 2004
Printed in the United States of America

⊛ The paper used in this publication meets the requirements of
the American National Standard for Information Sciences—Permanence
of Paper for Printed Library Materials, ANSI Z39.48-1984

Library of Congress Cataloging-in-Publication Data
Elson, Jean, 1948–
    Am I still a woman? : hysterectomy and gender identity / Jean Elson.
        p.   cm.
    Includes bibliographical references and index.
    ISBN 1-59213-210-3 (cloth : alk. paper) — ISBN 1-59213-211-1 (pbk. :
alk. paper)
        1. Women—Identity. 2. Hysterectomy—Psychological aspects.
    3. Hysterectomy—Patients—Psychology. 4. Body, Human—Social aspects.
    I. Title.
    HQ1206.E45 2004
    305.4—dc21

                                                                2003050787

Excerpt on page 1 from "In Celebration of My Uterus," from *Love Poems* by
Anne Sexton. Copyright © 1967, 1968, 1969 by Anne Sexton. Reprinted by
permission of Houghton Mifflin Company. All rights reserved.

2 4 6 8 9 7 5 3 1

Contents

098934953

3 1544

Acknowledgments

There are two ways of spreading light:
To be the candle or the mirror that receives it.

—*Edith Wharton*

I DEDICATE this book to my family, whose belief that I would reach my goal, enthusiasm for my project, and encouragement during difficult times has never wavered. My parents, Edith and Matthew Elson, have given me both roots and wings. I cannot fully articulate what their guidance has meant to my life and my work. My children, Gabriel David Poznik and Jessica Elson Poznik, have inspired me to live up to their pride in me and have grown into individuals of whom I am intensely proud.

I also dedicate my work to two grandmothers—Jenny, who never knew me but for whom I am named, and Bessie, who knew me quite well. Her aphorism, "Nothing but trying," echoed in my head throughout the challenging undertaking of pursuing and completing a Ph.D. at mid-life. These grandmothers exemplify the many "unknown" women who Virginia Woolf describes as having "been before me, making the path smooth, and regulating my steps."

This book began as a doctoral dissertation at Brandeis University. I am especially indebted to the support of my intellectual big brother and sister, Peter Conrad and Shulamit Reinharz. In addition to welcoming me to medical sociology, Peter motivated me to do my best work and gave me the confidence to know that I could. Shula is a wonderful teacher, friend, and mentor, and she kept me faithful to a feminist vision of this project. Many thanks also to Stefan Timmermans, and to Catherine Kohler Riessman for her active participation on my dissertation committee as well as for representing an important role model as a feminist medical sociologist. Furthermore, I could not have undertaken this project without the example of the pioneer women's health scholars I cite throughout this book.

I am grateful to the members of my dissertation writing group. Cameron MacDonald and Henry Rubin contributed many important insights to the early stages of my work, and Faith Ferguson deserves special mention. I extend my great appreciation to the Brandeis National Women's Committee, whose hard work has helped establish the Brandeis University Libraries as substantial scholarly resources.

Barry Elson is a brother in the very best sense, and his example gives me faith in the positive potential of the medical profession. Good friends, most notably Jayna Kraslin and Kathy Hart, have helped me negotiate the twists and turns that my professional and personal lives have taken over the last several years. Thanks also for the encouragement from colleagues and students in the Department of Sociology at the University of New Hampshire.

I express my gratitude to Michael Ames for his original interest and endorsement of this book project, and to Janet Francendese for her continued support and excellent editorial direction. Dr. Lucy Candib, of Worcester City Hospital, was an important source for referrals of minority and low income respondents. Credit is also due to Cherie Potts, whose transcription skills made my work so much easier.

I gratefully acknowledge the many generous sources of financial support that I received toward the completion of my graduate studies and my dissertation. This included scholarships and fellowships from the Brandeis University Graduate School of Arts and Sciences, as well as the Graduate Grant Prize for Research in Women's Studies from the Women's Studies Program at Brandeis.

I also appreciate the 1999 Graduate Student Paper award presented to me by the Division of Health, Health Policy, and Health Services of the Society for the Study of Social Problems, which encouraged me early on. I was greatly honored by the award of The Elizabeth Stanton Michaels Fellowship from the national American Association of University Women (AAUW), which provided me with both substantial funds and motivation to complete my dissertation.

Finally, I thank my most important resources for this project—the forty-four anonymous women who shared their time, their experiences, and their insights. Each interview was extremely valuable to my work, and every one of them is represented in my analysis. Respondents and I laughed and cried together, and perhaps even found a core of sisterhood, despite external differences. As always, I am impressed by the extraordinary wisdom that emanates from supposedly "ordinary" women.

1

"To Have and Have Not"

Perspectives on Hysterectomy and Oophorectomy

Everyone in me is a bird.
I am beating all my wings.
They wanted to cut you out
but they will not.
They said you were immeasurably empty
but you are not.
They said you were sick unto dying
but they were wrong.

You are singing like a school girl.
You are not torn.
Sweet weight,
in celebration of the woman I am
and of the soul of the woman I am
and of the central creature and its delight
I sing for you. I dare to live.
Hello, spirit. Hello, cup.
Fasten, cover. Cover that does contain.
Hello to the soil of the fields.
Welcome, roots . . .

—*Anne Sexton, "In Celebration of My Uterus"*

THESE LINES celebrate the poet's relief at discovering that she will not have to undergo hysterectomy, the surgical removal of her uterus. The rest of the poem celebrates womanhood in many forms. Appropriately included in a collection entitled *Love*

1

Poems, it expresses a woman's love for a valued part of her self. According to another feminist poet, this poem "finds unity where the culture propagates division: between a woman's sexuality and her spirituality, her creativity and her procreativity, herself and other women, her private and public self" (Ostriker 1986, 111).

The *uterus* is a woman's womb, which contains and nourishes a fetus during gestation. Most women also have two *ovaries,* which produce *ova* (eggs) and sex hormones. The normal nonpregnant human uterus weighs only approximately two ounces and is merely three inches long; the ovaries are even tinier, only one inch by one and a half inches. However, these sexual/reproductive organs carry great cultural and personal significance.

Most women do not consider the meanings of their uteruses and ovaries until they are faced with a crisis, as was Ann Sexton, whose poem is cited at the beginning of this chapter. In this book I explore the experiences of forty-four American women who have undergone hysterectomy (surgical removal of the uterus), with or without oophorectomy (surgical removal of the ovary), for benign conditions. Hysterectomy and oophorectomy offer women a unique opportunity to contemplate the meaning of their sexual reproductive organs in the context of female identity. One respondent described this crisis:

> I never really thought about having a uterus and ovaries until they were gone. After surgery, I wondered what it meant to be without those body parts—I mean, I'm really confused, I don't really know—"Am I still a woman?" (Janet)

Her words highlight the potential challenge to gender identity that is the major theme of my research . I explore how—whether they perceived loss, stability, or enhancement—respondents dealt with possible contradictions in gender identity presented by absent sexual reproductive organs.

Definitions and Demographics of Hysterectomy

In popular (and even scholarly) usage, there is often confusion over precisely what body parts are removed during hysterectomy.[1]

In fact, one or both of a woman's ovaries may be left intact after hysterectomy unless she undergoes an additional surgery called *bilateral salpingo-oophorectomy* (bs-o), and her cervix may even remain following *subtotal hysterectomy.* Furthermore, the uterus may be removed through a variety of different types of hysterectomies. While abdominal surgery is currently the most common type, comprising 63 percent of all procedures, 23 percent are performed by the vaginal method; and vaginal laparoscopic hysterectomy now represents 10 percent of surgeries (Lepine et al. 1997). Table 1 (p. 4) indicates some medical definitions that help clarify the subject matter of this book.

A common belief that hysterectomy rates have decreased appreciably in the United States is not borne out by fact. Following criticisms regarding unnecessary hysterectomies, the annual rates of hysterectomies did decline moderately from 7.1 per 1,000 women in 1980 to 6.6 per 1,000 women in 1987. However, according to data from the Agency for Healthcare Quality, hysterectomy rates in the United States for noncancerous conditions changed little in the next decade—from 5.5 per 1,000 women in 1990 to 5.6 per 1,000 women in 1997 (Farquhar and Steiner 2002). This is despite the development of several new therapeutic techniques as alternatives to hysterectomy.[2]

Hysterectomy is currently the second most commonly performed surgical procedure in the United States.[3] Each year approximately 600,000 American women undergo hysterectomies, a rate that is among the world's highest—three to four times higher than in Australia, New Zealand, and almost all European countries (Farquhar and Steiner 2002). In fact, the uterus of at least one out of every three American women is eventually surgically removed, and approximately 75 percent of these surgeries are performed on women between the ages of 20 and 49, most of who are premenopausal.[4] These statistics have remained constant over the last twenty years (Rock and Thompson 1997), though rates vary widely within the United States (nearly twice as high in the South as in the Northeast, for example) (Lepine et al. 1997).

Unlike mastectomies, most hysterectomies and oophorectomies are not performed to save lives: surgeries to treat cancer of

TABLE 1   Medical Definitions of Gynecological Surgery

Name	Alternative Names and Abbreviations	Definition
Subtotal hysterectomy	Partial hysterectomy Supracervical hysterectomy	Surgical removal of the *fundus* (body of the uterus)
Total abdominal hysterectomy	TAH	Abdominal surgical removal of the entire uterus, including both the *fundus* and the *cervix* (the neck of the uterus, which projects into the vagina and opens to release menstrual blood and to give birth)
Total vaginal hysterectomy	TVH	Surgical removal of the entire uterus, including both the *fundus* and the *cervix*, through the vagina
Laparoscopic assisted vaginal hysterectomy	LAVH TLH	Vaginal hysterectomy with visualization and resection of the uterine ligaments through a laparoscope that is inserted near the umbilicus, with the uterus removed through the vagina
Oophorectomy	Ovariotomy Ovarectomy Ovariectomy	Surgical removal of the ovary
Salpingo-oophorectomy		Surgical removal of the ovary and the connected *fallopian tube* (where the egg is fertilized and transported to the uterus)
Bilateral salpingo-oophorectomy	bs-o	Surgical removal of both fallopian tubes and both ovaries
Total hysterectomy–bilateral salpingo-oophorectomy	TAH-BSO TVH-BSO TLH-BSO	Removal of the entire uterus, both fallopian tubes, and both ovaries

the uterus, cervix, or ovaries account for only 10 percent of the total (Angier 1997; Franklin 1991). The most frequent reasons for hysterectomies and/or oophorectomies are for benign (though many times painful and annoying) conditions, including fibroid cysts, also known as leiomyomas (30 percent); endometriosis (20 percent); adenomyosis, sustained heavy bleeding (20 percent); pelvic inflammatory disease, genital prolapse (15 percent); and unexplained chronic pelvic pain (10 percent) (Brody 1993). Although the majority of hysterectomies and oophorectomies are considered "elective" because they are done for reasons that are not life threatening, it is unclear how much choice women actually have, since they are seldom privy to diverse and accurate information regarding these surgeries and alternatives (Lippert 1993). In fact, researchers have found that at least one-third of all American hysterectomies are probably "medically unnecessary" (Franklin 1991). Furthermore, according to the U.S. Centers for Disease Control and Prevention, healthy ovaries are also removed during a large proportion of hysterectomies (Angier 1997).

Michel Foucault's work reinforces the extent to which "our bodies are trained, shaped, and impressed with the stamp of prevailing historical forms of selfhood, desire, masculinity, femininity" (Bordo 1993, 165–66). Long historical precedent associates women's gender identities with their sexual reproductive organs; uteruses and ovaries have even been employed as a synecdoche for women in their entirety (Laqueur 1990).[5] In fact, according to *New York Times* science reporter Natalie Angier, some medical sources claim that the uterus is "the only part of the body that is unique to women, the one organ that doesn't have an anatomical equivalent in the male" (1999, 84).[6] Hence, these body parts hold the potential to serve as "symbolic resources which facilitate interpretation" (cf. Olesen et al. 1990, 453) of cultural conceptions regarding female biology and feminine gender identity.[7] The theory that uteruses and ovaries constitute the core of women's gender identity implies that without these organs an individual may not be considered female. Accordingly, Wolf (1970, 165) depicts hysterectomy as "a surgical disruption to the self-concept of 'femininity' due to the central role of the uterus in the development of women's perspectives regarding body image, social role, and gender role. Women who have undergone hysterectomy may consequently see themselves as defeminised by having a hysterectomy."

Gender Identity

Although Goffman's claim that "gender, not religion, is the opiate of the masses" may be somewhat extreme, his contention that gender identity involves "the deepest sense of what one is" reflects an important social fact (1977, 315). While it is fashionable in some academic circles to insist that gender identity no longer matters, this is not the case in the real world. As Lynne Segal observes, "The idea that we are, or may soon become, post-gender exists alongside the continuing potency of the narrative of basic gender polarity" (2000, 120).

Many social theorists assert that gender identity is one of the most fundamental means by which individuals are recognized, both by others and by themselves. According to one scholar, "People may be described and categorized along many dimensions, but few seem to be as salient as gender. . . . [G]ender is an integral part of who were are, how we think about ourselves, and how others respond to us" (Katz 1979, 155). Another theorist concludes, "Being female or being male is a part of everyone's social identity from birth till death. Gender is at the core of what we 'really are'" (Stoll 1974, ix).

While gender is a primary identity for everyone, it may be particularly salient for women. For example, Deaux and Major (1990, 93) found that women are more likely to spontaneously describe themselves by gender than are men. Although many social theorists claim that gender is a crucial component of identity, there is disagreement as to what actually constitutes gender. Theories regarding gender generally begin with the assumption that biology, socialization, or social construction takes precedence. Either "anatomy is destiny," or social factors make biology moot. For clarity,

I will briefly summarize various theories of gender and then explain the approach that I find most reasonable.

Biological Essentialist Theories

The sociological concept of essentialism stems from philosophical arguments dating back to Aristotle that things, including people, have essences—necessary properties that make them what they are. The term *sex* has been related to the "natural" biological category of woman (or man), while *gender* has been connected to culturally produced processes. Biological essentialists generally believe that sex is inborn and that gender is the social manifestation of sex. According to this schema, there can only be two bipolar sexes and two bipolar genders. Sex can either be male or female; gender can only be masculine or feminine. According to most feminist analyses, biological essence is a conservative strategy often used as an excuse to sustain and fortify differences in male and female roles (e.g., de Beauvoir 1976; Friedan 1963; Millet 1970; Firestone 1970; Greer 1970). Nevertheless, several radical feminists have appropriated the concept of essence to argue that women's essential nature is more prosocial than men's (e.g. Snitow 1990; Ruddick 1989; Rich 1986a; Rossi 1977; Mitchell 1973). These theorists assert that patriarchal (male-dominated) society has alienated women from their essential nature, which should be strengthened, rather than minimized. Despite strong arguments from both sides of the political spectrum, a number of social scientists (e.g., Connell 1987; Deaux and Kite 1987; Epstein 1988; Lorber 1994) and biological scientists (e.g., Bleier 1984; Fausto-Sterling 1985; 1987; 1993; Hubbard, Henifen, and Fried 1977) have critiqued the biological essentialist model of gender by describing the circular process by which purportedly objective and natural understandings of sex are actually shaped by social influences.

Cultural Essentialist Theories

Sex role or socialization theories of gender view society and nature as additive. They assert that the "natural" dichotomy between genders is clarified through cultural elaboration. While the biological essentialist position emphasizes that gender behavior is inherently tied to sex, sex role or socialization theory maintains that gender is learned through an individual's developing understanding of what characteristics and behaviors are considered culturally acceptable for individuals who are born either male or female (Howard and Hollander 1997).

Although socialization theories connect social structure to personality formation, they generally rely on stereotyped interpersonal expectations that do not explain the association between personal agency and social structure (Connell 1987). Like biological essentialist theory, sex role or socialization theories still define gender in terms of dichotomous difference. Males or females are expected to enact only one of two gendered roles, the "masculine" or the "feminine." Accordingly, social gender is no more flexible than biological sex, and socialization or sex role theory may be interpreted as a form of cultural essentialism.

Social Constructionist Theories

In general, the social constructionist position on gender, founded on symbolic interaction, maintains that gender is created through interpersonal interpretation of action. The insight that gender identity is not just something a person *is*, but is produced through performance, has origins in the work of Erving Goffman (1977), who focuses on "gender displays" as highly conventionalized behaviors that are situational rather than ongoing. Social constructionists expand this concept to assert that gender is an emergent feature of social situations rather than a property of individuals (West and Zimmerman 1987).

Ethnomethodology is a form of social construction that is particularly useful for examining social phenomena by analyzing how "irreducible facts" accepted by members of a shared culture are actually beliefs produced through social interaction. Harold Garfinkel (1967), the founder of ethnomethodology, used a case study of "Agnes," a transsexual, to demonstrate that gender is accomplished through everyday behavior. Agnes was able to convince people that she was a woman by learning to enact "womanly" mannerisms, dress, and behavior. Garfinkel maintained that Agnes's strategies of self-presentation are entirely comparable to the strategies employed by "normal" females, which are so taken for granted that they are invisible.

Building on the ethnomethodological approach, Suzanne Kessler and Wendy McKenna claim that a "gender attribution" (the decision whether an individual is either male or female) is made every time we see a new person. Furthermore, they argue, "The 'decision' that we make as to whether that person is a man or a woman is not stated in terms of probabilities." People are considered to be "either one or the other, zero or 100 percent" (1978, 2). Despite the fact that there is considerable individual variation in characteristics, gender is commonly attributed as bipolar rather than as a continuum of possibilities. "It is only by questioning dichotomous criteria for gender attributions," Kessler and McKenna claim, "that the dichotomous nature of gender, itself, becomes problematic" (12). According to these sociologists, gender identity "refers to an individual's own feeling of whether she or he is a woman or a man, or a girl or a boy. In essence gender identity is self-attribution of gender" (8). Kessler and McKenna propose that people do not always follow the same rules when attributing gender to self and to others. However, they assert that it is difficult for an individual to maintain a self-image without a clear gender identity.

Kessler and McKenna are among the growing number of social theorists who argue that not only gender but also the bipolar categories of biological sex are socially constructed (see also Scott 1988). According to this theoretical position, "society not only shapes personality and behavior, it also shapes the ways in which the body appears. But if the body is itself always seen through social interpretation, then sex is not something that is separate from gender, but is, rather, that which is subsumable under it" (Nicholson 1994, 79).

Gender is presumably assigned to people based on their genitals, internal organs, or chromosomes. Nonetheless, gender attributions in everyday life are made, not by undressing people or by administering physical exams or laboratory tests, but through observing cultural factors of behavior, dress, mannerisms, and so forth. Therefore, biological theories of gender actually rely on the social process of gender attribution. Social constructionists consider gender to be an emergent feature of social situations rather than a property of individuals. As empirical proof, Kessler and McKenna (1978) discuss examples of individuals who illuminate the social rules regarding gender through transgression of these rules. These include transsexuals, intersexuals, and other individuals with unusual chromosomal and hormonal characteristics. My intention in undertaking the current study was to explore the phenomenon of gender identity by studying individuals who have undergone surgical removal of their uteruses (hysterectomy) and/or their ovaries (oophorectomy), a far more ordinary experience than the examples employed by Kessler and McKenna.

Based on their analysis that sex is subordinate to gender, Kessler and McKenna (1978) employ the term *gender* even when discussing biological differences. Meredith Kimball also recommends using *gender* as a general term to emphasize that all differences, even if based in biology, are socially constructed: "The use of gender is to remind myself and the reader that any particular difference or similarity is the result of complex and sometimes contradictory social processes that involve individuals, social institutions, and cultural beliefs" (1995, 18–19; see also Deaux 1993; Unger and Crawford 1993). Since I consider this an appropriate practice, I refer to *gender identity* rather than *sex identity* throughout this book.

Performance Theories

The performance theory of gender developed by philosopher Judith Butler is somewhat compatible with the social constructionist perspective in sociology. Butler (1993) denies that the formulation of gender is the cultural interpretation of sex; rather, she believes that sex is produced and established through cultural discourses. In addition, she emphasizes that the subject who becomes a woman is not necessarily biologically female. According to her theory, gender does not follow naturally from sex; "naturalization" is a difficult and continuing process and can be confirmed only through repeated performance. For Butler, gender is never a stable identity but is always a process of becoming, and sex is not a given but an "artificial unity" imposed on "an otherwise discontinuous set of attributes" (1993, 114). As Jennifer Harding points out, "The notion of performance fits more closely with popular cultural perceptions that femininity is an elusive ideal which must be constantly sought but never attained, and with some feminist descriptions of femininity as an identity in process, never complete" (1998, 3).

Toward a Synthesis of Theories about Gender

As I delineate in later chapters, the women that I interviewed struggled with their own lay versions of biological essentialist, sex role, social construction, and performance theories. While I find social constructionist theory the most useful approach to studying gender identity, this perspective does not entirely describe the experience of living in a biological body. Robert Connell (1987) is one of several social theorists who warn against emphasizing the social aspects of gender to the point of minimizing the importance of the material body. It is crucial to bear in mind that an individual develops her sense of identity from perceptions received through her body and expresses her identity through her body. Yet as Elizabeth Spelman (1988) aptly points out, feminist sociology has tended to be particularly "somatophobic" because women's bodies have been the basis for biological determinism. As I will demonstrate throughout this book, respondents' experiences indicate that the biological essentialist position, which associates sexual reproductive organs with the essence of being a woman, is highly problematic. However, this does not mean that ovaries and uteruses have nothing to do with gender identity, as other respondents discuss. The women I interviewed continuously cross back and forth between the boundaries of woman as sex (biology) and as gender (social and cultural prescriptions).

Other social theorists articulate a position that synthesizes seemingly disparate perspectives regarding gender. "In and of itself, essentialism is neither good nor bad, progressive nor reactionary, beneficial nor dangerous," Diana Fuss (1989, xi) proposes. She further argues that there is no clear distinction between essentialist and social constructionist discourses. According to her, constructionism is actually only "a more sophisticated form of essentialism" (xii). She maintains that, while constructionists challenge the historicity of essentialism, they also "often work with uncomplicated or essentializing notions of history. While a constructionist might recognize that *man* and *woman* are produced across a spectrum of discourses, the categories *man* and *woman* still remain constant" (3). According to this rationale, social constructionist theories must incorporate essentialism.

Sociologists Simon Williams and Gillian Bendelow examine the claims of essentialism and social construction and propose a "third stage of conceptual development" (1998, 3). They suggest that the term *embodiment* provides the means for partially transcending the "nature vs. culture" debate. Williams and Bendelow argue the need for an "embodied sociology" that would shift from theorizing *about* bodies in a disembodied manner to perspectives of theorizing *from* lived bodies. They therefore call for a move "towards a more integrated social theory of embodiment—one that links (lived) *experience* to (cultural) *representation*" (1998, 3). This is compatible with Adrienne Rich's suggestion that feminists remind ourselves that the body is not only an abstract construct but also a material fact of life (1986b, 215). Since I agree with these theorists, this book emphasizes personal embodied experience over universal theories of bodies.

Helen Marshall advocates that a phenomenological approach is fundamental to theorizing the body and expresses concern that "so much attention is being paid to nomenclature and theory, and so little to the lived experiences and data" (1996, 255). In order to understand the lived experiences of respondents, I have recognized that respondents inhabit real bodies, not just cultural representations of bodies. The pain that they feel, both physical and emotional, is authentic. As a sociologist, I view the social environment as crucial; and accordingly, paying attention to the biological body does not mean that I endorse biological reductionism. I support Susan Bordo's contention that the female body is "*both* construction *and* resource" (1993, 36). My goal is to understand the complicated interaction between body and society in order to interpret respondents' experiences. To rely exclusively on one particular theory of gender would "turn what is valuable as a partial vision into a flawed whole" (Kimball 1995, 1). The perspective from which I have analyzed and interpreted respondents' interviews is thus that *the body is not totally constructed by social discourse or socialization processes, nor does it exist completely independently of these.*

To paraphrase Steven Epstein (1990, 286), "Neither strict constructionism nor strict essentialism are capable of [fully] explaining what it means to be [a woman]." *Woman* is at the same time an "empty" and "overflowing" category (Lorber 1994; Scott 1988); it can represent biology, socialization, role performance, or discourse. In this book, I apply the term *woman* to both sex and gender. Since respondents used the term in each of these ways, I reflect their multiple meanings of *woman* in my analysis. I hope to further the theoretical move toward reconciling the materiality and social construction of women's bodies.

Biographical Disruption of Gender Identity

My research and analysis employs the *experience of illness perspective* within medical sociology, which focuses on subjective understanding of what it is like to have a medical condition (see Conrad 1987; Fitzpatrick et al. 1984; Schneider and Conrad 1983). The chronic conditions of having undergone hysterectomy and oophorectomy fit Conrad's definition of "lived-with illnesses" because people must adapt and learn to live with them, but they are not (usually) life-threatening. This is similar to Greil's (1991a; 1991b) contention that the condition of infertility can be seen as comparable to chronic illness.

Medical events often generate *biographical disruptions* or *turning points;* the individual's concept of who she or he is will never be the same as before.[8] Bryan Turner maintains that a sociology of the body allows medical sociologists to appreciate "the intimate and necessary relationship between my sense of myself, my awareness of the integrity of my body and experience of illness as not simply an attack on my instrumental body *(körper)* but as a radical intrusion into my embodied selfhood" (1992, 167). Accordingly, "to change our embodiment is to change our identity" (256). Turner's work is foundational for my specific project of examining the effects of gynecological surgery on gender identity.

Michael Bury (1982, 169) conceptualizes chronic illness as "a major kind of disruptive experience, or, using Anthony Giddens (1979) term, 'critical situation.'" Bury connects three aspects of disruption to chronic illness: disruption of taken-for-granted assumptions and behaviors; more profound disruptions in explanatory systems that cause an individual to rethink her or his own biography and self-concept; and finally, the necessary mobilization of resources to face the crisis in identity. A similar concept is found in Juliet Corbin and Anselm Strauss's concept of *turning points* in chronic illness (1985, 1987). Turning points are seen as critical incidents that force individuals to recognize that their lives have changed in crucial ways and that they will have to reevaluate and revise their former assumed identities (Strauss 1959). Turning points may be met with a diversity of emotional reactions and coping strategies.

Kathy Charmaz has done some of the most interesting work regarding the impact of chronic conditions on identity. In several articles (1983; 1987; 1990; 1994; 1999a; 1999b) and her book (1991), she employs the symbolic interactionist perspective to discover the ways in which physical diversity can result in a "loss of self." Virginia Olesen and her co-authors observe that even minor bodily disturbances such as a rash can cause sufferers to alter their views of themselves. They argue that people who suffer more severe bodily changes through surgery (i.e., ostomates) do not merely see changed images of their bodies; they perceive themselves as "transformed beings whose physical and social capacities had been substantially altered" (Olesen et al. 1990, 452). All of this sociological research supports my specific project of examining the effects of hysterectomy and/or oophorectomy on gender identity.

Brief Historical Background of Hysterectomy and Oophorectomy

Hysterectomy and oophorectomy constitute surgeries that have long histories. Throughout differing time periods, the significance of wombs and ovaries and the effect of these gynecological surgeries on the perception of an individual's *womanhood* have been interpreted very differently.

Prior to empirical studies about the effects of oophorectomy and hysterectomy, a variety of cultural theories proposed the importance of female reproductive organs. For example, the ancient Egyptians and Greeks attributed women's supposed emotional instability to a "wandering womb." In fact, the root of the term *hysteria* derives from the Greek word *hyster,* meaning womb. Hippocrates theorized that the human uterus had numerous chambers and was lined with "tentacles" or "suckers," an erroneous belief that persisted until the Renaissance, due to prohibitions regarding dissection of the human body (Angier 1999). Surgery to remove the uterus was apparently accomplished in ancient times, with the first recorded hysterectomy performed by the Greek physician Arhigenes in A.D. 100. Vaginal hysterectomy was the traditional way to remove the uterus in antiquity.

Notions that the womb dominated the female body in ways that could cause a woman to go mad continued well into the nineteenth century. As the concept of the body as an organism gave way to a view of the body as a machine during the nineteenth century, female bodies were found particularly defective and in need of repair. The growing profession of gynecology appropriated primary responsibility for the female body (Barker-Benfield 1976). Ovariotomies were first performed in the early nineteenth century for the purpose of removing huge ovarian tumors. Later, surgeries to excise ovaries were no longer limited to purely medical rationales. The belief that the reproductive organs completely controlled women's bodies and minds between puberty and menopause provoked their removal for a wide variety of reasons.[9] Victorian physicians insisted that the "instability of their reproductive systems interfered with [women's] sexual, emotional, and rational control" (Showalter 1987, 55). Removing healthy female organs was seen as necessary in order to cure the "so-called failures of femininity"(Laqueur 1990, 176), which included "ovariomania," "hystero-epilepsy," nymphomania, masturbation, suicidal tendencies, dysmenorrhea, overeating, and many other physical and psychological symptoms. After the advent of anesthesia in the nineteenth century, abdominal hysterectomy surpassed vaginal hysterectomy as the predominant method of removing the uterus.[10] As hysterectomy became a medically safer operation, it replaced *ovariotomy* as a "cure" for a variety of women's presumed physiological and psychological problems, most notably hysteria and melancholia (an early concept of depression). Physicians continued to perform this surgery despite the fact that out of 400 hysterectomies from 1881 to 1885, there was a 50 percent death rate (Dally 1991, 220).

Finally, at the turn of the twentieth century, members of the medical community began to denounce the practice of widespread *normal ovariotomy*, the surgical removal of the ovaries for other than physical problems (Dally 1991). Eventually, normal ovariotomy was banned in many places, and surgeons who performed it were referred to as "belly-rippers." Some historical researchers assert that the medical profession condemned gynecological surgery performed for psychological and behavioral rationales primarily because it failed the objective of inducing women to conform to their expected gender roles (see Barker-Benfield 1976). The current medical assumption is that hysterectomies and oophorectomies are performed solely for physical problems, although this is not always the case (Bernstein et al. 1997).

Previous Scholarly Research

Although feminist sociologists have conducted extensive research on the lived experiences of "natural" menopause (e.g., Bell 1987; Kaufert 1982; Rogers 1997), they have not sufficiently explored the experiences of women who reach this stage through surgery. With the exception of my own work on the subject, previous sociological discussions regarding hysterectomy have focused almost entirely on this surgery as an example of medical misogyny and social control (e.g., Fisher 1986, Scully 1994).[11] While this is an important aspect, the removal of sexual reproductive organs can also present an opportunity to provide insight into the relationship between cultural and lived experiences of the gendered body. Given the frequency with which women undergo hysterectomy and the removal of their ovaries (oophorectomy), it is surprising that sociologists have not previously conducted more sophisticated analyses of the impact these surgeries may have on the social construction of gender identity.

Medical doctors, nurses, and psychologists have conducted the overwhelming majority of studies on psychosocial outcomes of oophorectomy and hysterectomy, both prospective and retrospective. Major difficulties that arise in comparing previous studies regarding women's experiences with hysterectomy include dissimilar methodologies: large variations in measures of emotional symptoms, length of follow-up, and wording of survey questions (Bernstein et al. 1997). Findings from these studies vary widely, with estimates of the proportion of women suffering from postoperative psychological problems ranging from 4 percent to 66 percent (Bernstein et al. 1997). This impedes definitive conclusions.

Much of the medical and psychological research does indicate that women may suffer negative emotional outcomes as a result of hysterectomy, particularly related to feelings of the loss of femininity.[12] For example, according to Polivy, "a threat to [sexual/reproductive organs] can easily constitute a threat to a woman's whole self-concept" (1974, 417). Correspondingly, Kaltreider, Wallace, and Horowitz (1979) claim that depression and other negative psychological consequences following hysterectomy are prompted by a major negative alteration in an individual's internal image of herself as a woman. Webb and Wilson-Barnett found: "A review of over sixty articles in medical journals suggests that women recovering from hysterectomy may find their image of themselves radically changed even though there is no visible alteration in the body. For some women, having a hysterectomy may pose a profound threat to their self-concept as a feminine person, an attractive sexual being for whom childbearing has been a major and highly valued social role" (1983, 97). However, in their own study, these researchers did not find that self-concept was damaged. A primary objective of this book is to investigate whether respondents do experience this loss to gender identity, and if so, specifically how it is manifested.

While many previous studies show that women experience negative identity consequences, other medical and psychological research finds that women do *not* suffer losses to their gender identities as a result of gynecological surgery. Several studies assert that subjects' feelings regarding their gender identities are not changed in any way by hysterectomy.[13] Even more surprising in light of other studies showing negative emotional outcomes, some medical and psychological research claims that women experience marked *improvement* in mood after hysterectomy.[14] I also examine this proposition, particularly since these studies do not fully explore the reasons behind reported neutral or positive emotional effects.

Some medical and psychological research attempts to establish that women who undergo hysterectomy have a history of previous psychosocial problems prior to surgery,[15] but these studies do not adequately explain the reasons for this connection. These researchers may be practicing an unfounded "blaming the victim" that implies that women's depression may actually cause them to seek hysterectomies. The inherent assumption in these studies is that depression is the independent variable. However, as described in the following chapters, my research demonstrates that many women endure extended periods of heavy bleeding and intense pain prior to finally undergoing hysterectomies. It is more likely that this physical suffering is the independent variable that causes psychological symptoms prior to surgery and is also the medical reason for hysterectomy. Earlier studies on hysterectomy include several major weaknesses. First, the most prominent research (Cosper, Fuller, and Robinson 1978; Drelich and Bieber 1958; Hampton and Tarnasky 1974; Kaltreider, Wallace, and Horowitz 1979; Patterson and Craig 1963; Polivy 1974; B. Richards 1978; D. Richards 1974: Webb and Wilson-Barnett 1983) was conducted many years ago, whereas both scholarly and lay conceptions of gender have changed considerably since then. Second, previous researchers generally neglected to separate out the effects of hysterectomy (removal of the uterus) for women who retained their ovaries and those who did not. Another important problem with most scholarly work is the researchers' assumptions that women's reactions to gynecological surgery are uniform, despite differing social factors such as age and menopausal status at the time of surgery, desire for (more) children, significant emotional and sexual relationships, and the personal salience of gender identity. Finally, most previous studies did not make use of intensive interviewing in order to focus on the lived experiences of women who have undergone these surgeries (Ryan 1997).

Self-Help Discourse

A proliferation of self-help literature regarding women's health issues has been stimulated by the women's health movement (Zimmerman 1987). As Allwood (1996) points out, "The self-help genre is one that has been mainly directed towards women, and provides a site to examine contested notions of expertise and responsibility in a specific area" (qtd. in Lyons and Griffin 2000, 470). Self-help books on hysterectomy and oophorectomy generally include detailed descriptions of the experiences of women who have undergone these surgeries.

I have reviewed seventeen self-help books regarding hysterectomy.[16] These books are sometimes intended to offer advice to women who have already had hysterectomies but are most often written for an audience facing the possibility of future surgery.[17] The titles of many of these books—for example, *No More Hysterectomies* (Hufnagel 1988); *Male Practice: How Doctors Manipulate Women* (Mendelsohn 1981); *You Don't Need a Hysterectomy* (Strausz 1993); *The Castrated Woman: What Your Doctor Won't Tell You About Hysterectomy* (Stokes 1986); *The Ultimate Rape: What Every Woman Should Know About Hysterectomies and Ovarian Removal* (Plourde 1998)—generally reflect the concept that gynecological surgery is to be avoided at all costs. A common opening line from one of these self-help books reads: "In this book I will give you ammunition to defend yourself against hysterectomy" (West 1994, 13).

Self-help books include narratives from women who have undergone or were spared from undergoing hysterectomy or oophorectomy. These narratives are often framed as cautionary tales, including "winners" (those who kept their sexual reproductive organs, and in several examples even got pregnant) and "losers" (those who lost their uteruses and/or ovaries). In most triumphant accounts, a woman combats a member of the medical establishment in order to save herself. She becomes a "winner" either by resisting surgery herself or being saved by, or with the help of, another individual, usually a "white knight" husband or enlightened physician. The discussion of gynecological surgery in terms of informed decision making is especially striking. These books offer a form of resistance and thus provide an alternative discourse to medical discourse on gynecological surgery.

The "Hyster Sisters Recovery Web site" was launched in 1998 with the stated purpose of serving women who had either undergone or were anticipating hysterectomy. In 2001, a book based on the Web site was published; it was called *Through the Land of Hyster: The Hyster Sister Guide* (Kelley 2001). Similar to other self-help literature regarding hysterectomy, this Web site and book portray tales of survival and triumph over evil. However, contrary to the often gloomy tone of previous self-help books regarding hysterectomy outcomes, the narratives are generally lighter in tone, tongue-in-cheek, and even somewhat flippant. The founder of the site, Kathy Kelley (the "Keeper of the Book"), created a "Land of Hyster, with a wonderful King and the land full of loving Hyster Sisters: Ladies in Waiting [those women anticipating hysterectomy] and Punctured Princesses [those women who have already undergone hysterectomy]." Women who contribute to the site are referred to either as Princess [name] or Lady [name], and describe themselves as having previously visited "the Land of Ablation," "the Land of Hormones," or "the Land of Pap." The gender themes inherent in this self-help discourse are quite apparent, including an appeal to patriarchal authority (the King) and attempts to reclaim femininity.[18]

Self-help narratives provide a very real attempt to capture women's own perceptions of their experiences, including possible inconsistencies and contradictions. However, such literature is generally written with a political, rather than a scholarly intent and is uninformed by theoretical analysis.[19]

Previous Qualitative Research

Qualitative research enables a scholarly study of lived experiences. According to Murray and Chamberlain: "Qualitative research provides insights into individual perspectives that are rendered invisible in the aggregation which typifies quantitative approaches (Griffin and Phoenix 1994), providing space for the description and interpretation of subjective experience. This is particularly important for women's health where historically men have conducted the majority of health research" (2000, 43).

Several previous studies have used qualitative research methods, notably interviews, in order to study women's experiences of gynecological surgery.[20] However, since the existing research is based in either medical or psychological frameworks, it does not include comprehensive sociological perspectives, nor does it investigate the meanings of the diverse gender implications of gynecological surgery. In contrast, I intend this book to make use of the sociological imagination in order to explore the effects of hysterectomy and oophorectomy on gender identity.

The Research Method for This Book

My research goal in this study was to further elucidate the complicated interaction between the material body and the social body as elaborated by respondents' lived experiences with gynecological surgery. I chose to examine the impact of lost body parts on gender identity by studying women who had undergone surgery on sexual reproductive organs rather than by studying women who had undergone breast surgery for two reasons. First, although women who undergo mastectomy may also suffer problems with gender identity, the preponderance of these women also face a deadly disease. I was particularly interested in interviewing women for whom cancer was not a complicating factor. As previously mentioned, the vast majority of women who experience hysterectomies and oophorectomies are not suffering from cancer, and I interviewed only respondents who had undergone surgery for benign conditions. Second, the absence of a breast may be obvious to others, while uteruses and ovaries are seen as "hidden" body parts. This enabled me to interrogate the meanings that absence of these organs had for women as a *discreditable* vs. *discredited* stigma (Goffman 1963).

Since I was interested in women's lived experiences, an ethnographic research method was most suitable for my purpose. I chose to use the *grounded theory approach,* which discovers theory through the systematic collection, constant comparison, and analysis of interview data (Glaser and Strauss 1967). Grounded theory was particularly appropriate for my project since it is rooted in symbolic interaction and phenomenology. In addition to grounded theory, I also took advantage of *discourse analysis,* which looks at the role of language in the construction of reality, as well as "unplanned personal experience," data I encountered as part of everyday life (Reinharz 1992).

Forty-four women who had experienced hysterectomies for benign conditions participated in this project. As a result of my pilot study of ten women, I identified categories of respondent characteristics that I wanted to compare. Categories included age at surgery (ranging between 24 and 69, with a mean age of 38.9 years and a median age of 37.5); age at time of interview (ranging between 24 and 97); time interval since surgery (from nine weeks to sixty years); marital or partner status; sexual preference; parental status; and emergency or "elective" surgery status. While respondents comprised a convenience sample, I specifically sought to interview women who represented variations within these categories. In addition, I sought some racial and ethnic diversity, including mostly European American women, but also three African American women and five Latina Americans. (See the Appendix for more specific information about the respondents and the research methodology.)

The Diversity of Women's Experiences

I did not approach this research project with the expectation that very different women would react in the same ways simply because they underwent the same medical procedures. Nancy Tuana (1993) asserts that, while feminist standpoint theory reminds us that all knowledge arises out of experience, any feminist standpoint must necessarily be partial: "It cannot represent the experiences of 'woman,' because such a being does not exist." She warns that "there is a danger is expecting to find a common core of shared experiences, for such a quest will tend to blind us to the differences between women," and she suggests that "it is more realistic to expect pluralities of experiences that are related through various intersections or resemblances of some of the experiences of some women to some of the experiences of others" (Tuana 1993, 283). My in-depth interview methodology enabled me to uncover many of these inconsistencies and contradictions that are often obscured in quantitative studies. I have analyzed the intersections of respondents' experiences of hysterectomy and oophorectomy, noting that there are similarities as well as differences in these experiences. While I discuss these points in more detail in later chapters, the following interview excerpts provide an overview of respondents' answers to how surgery affected their feelings of gender identity, with the inherent question: "Am I still a woman?"

Some respondents expressed the belief that their identities as *women* were deeply affected in negative ways after hysterectomy:

> I felt useless. *I didn't feel like a woman.* . . . I'm not a woman. What makes a woman different from a man? (Margie)

> Ohhh, *I know I'm a woman, but I don't feel the same.* When I have my uterus, because that's part of my body. We grow with that part, every move I think is very difficult, very depressing for women . . . now I feel like a *fake woman.* (Isabella)

> I felt—I don't want to say 'violated', but *I feel like I'm not a whole woman any more* . . . just that, and you're missing something, you're lacking something that a woman should have. (Bernadette)

> Your menopause is a natural thing. . . . The menopause didn't bother me at all. . . . Because one was natural and the other wasn't. . . . *Just somehow you were no longer a woman* [following hysterectomy]. You know? (Deborah)

However, at least one respondent had some positive feelings about losing part of her female identity as a result of surgery:

> . . . *For the first time I got rid of all my women stuff and I was me.* (Alice)

A number of respondents reported that, although gynecological surgery prompted them to ponder the meanings of their uteruses and ovaries, they had ultimately concluded that their gender identities were secure:

> I am always; I have *always* been . . . the same person. That has not changed just because, a, an organ has been taken out of me, that hasn't changed me at all. . . . I feel womanly. . . . *Never, ever, ever felt any less of a woman.* (Joyce)

> *I never identified my uterus as identification of being a woman.* I always identified my uterus as a body organ. I think heterosexual women identify it as a part of their womanhood . . . is it because I'm a les-

bian? Or is it because I am who I am? I really don't know the answer to that. (Brooke)

And this whole bit about how you're no longer a woman because you don't (laughing). . . . I think that that's part of the socialization of how you feel about yourself as a person. And I think that the identity of an individual is a composite of a variety of things and sexuality and your being female is one piece of it. *And that I'm no less female because I don't have two ovaries.* That's not what identifies me as female. (Faye)

. . . *I never felt like I was less of a woman, ever.* (Wendy)

A cluster of respondents initially felt losses to their female identity, but over time, these women were able to reclaim their gender identities through forms of biographical work that I discuss in Chapter 7:

I'm all woman. . . . After the surgery I did feel like "Geeze. . . ." *I did feel a little of not being a complete woman any more.* . . . But it was very little. It lasted very little. (Lupe)

I felt for the first time in my life incomplete as a woman. . . . I never felt as though my reproductive organs complimented or completed me. But the absence thereof really was devastating. I really felt castrated. I really felt neutered in many ways . . . but my uterus and ovaries didn't make me who I am. Although at a time I really felt as though that defined my femininity and my womanhood. I never thought about them until they started giving me trouble. And I felt when they were taken from me and when I was trying to take care of them and they didn't respond and I truly lost them, that my womanhood or a part of my womanhood had been taken away. . . . *But that isn't what my womanhood is all about.* It's not some tissue with hormones in it that define who I am as a human being. There's much more than that emotionally and spiritually. . . . (Terry)

A final category of women felt that surgery made their gender identities even *more* secure than before:

. . . *If anything, my surgery has made me more of a woman.* Because it allowed me to enjoy myself as a woman [sexually]. (Page)

Well, at the time, it was incredibly traumatic and very surprising to me, that at some level I had bought into this biological determinism about my gender. . . . Well, I felt if I didn't have those parts and what made me female. . . . I think much more about me as a physical woman than I did before. . . . It's just that having that surgery was a big wake-up call for me, that I wasn't paying attention to my physical self and integrating that with my sense of my identity as a human being. . . . Initially, I felt really confused. What was I? *If I didn't have those parts, how could I be a woman?* . . . It sort of jolted me into an awareness that I needed to create a new paradigm for myself, that there wasn't one out there that I could just tap into. . . . *And this was a new opportunity for me to create my own definition of female identity, a woman's body.* And in that process I found myself becoming very, very empowered. (Andrea)

These divergent opinions affirm Lock's assertion that "the significance that an individual attributes to events is a cultural construct, but it is contextualized and interpreted in light of personal experience and inclination" (1993, 371). It is also important to note, as I discuss in following chapters, that individual rationales for change or stasis in female identity were variable. Moreover, many respondents are actually more ambivalent than these short excerpts demonstrate, sometimes making contrary statements and sometimes describing feelings and actions that conflict with their stated positions regarding female identity. I analyze these contradictions to the best of my sociological ability.

Preview of This Book

Implicit in descriptions of biographical disruption and turning point is the assumption that different individuals may suffer disparate degrees of disturbance from the same physical impetus. As I demonstrate throughout this book, some respondents believe that their bodies and lives were greatly altered by gynecological surgery, others sense very little change, and some perceive no change at all. However, for all forty-four respondents, hysterectomy and/or oophorectomy stimulated reflection regarding gender identity. According to Howard and Hollander, "Although everyone has a gender identity, the salience of this identity may vary among people" (1997, 16). This was certainly the case for respondents in my study.

Do respondents feel that surgical removal of their uteruses and/or ovaries has disrupted their gender identities to the extent that they are no longer women? Do they believe that they are still women due to a deeply innate essence? Do respondents maintain that they are still women because they perform feminine roles or appear outwardly feminine? Since for humans the social and biological are inseparable, decisions regarding identity are too complex to offer simplistic answers to these questions. Nevertheless, by paying close attention to respondents' experiences, I examined their nuanced understandings of the impact of surgery on their very personal perceptions of gender identity.

Some of the analytic messiness attached to my study stems from the contingency that respondents did not self-consciously seek gender identity transformations through surgery. This represents a very different situation from other sociological studies that examine the impact of surgery on gender identity. For example, individuals who undergo transsexual surgery read, talk, and think about the meanings of sex, sexuality, and gender before surgery. The vast majority of the women I interviewed were not theoretically sophisticated regarding sex and gender. Hysterectomy and oophorectomy were not chosen as the means to achieve new, desired gender identities, and, with few exceptions, prior to surgery they did not even have the opportunity to consider the meaning of either their sexual reproductive organs or their gender identity.

In this introductory chapter, I have explained definitions and demographics of hysterectomy and oophorectomy and clarified the concepts of gender identity and biographical disruption. I have contextualized this study by presenting a brief history of the association between sexual reproductive organs and the condition of *womanhood*. I have also briefly described previous research and the perspectives and methodologies that I used to analyze data from the interviews. In Chapters 2 and 3, I investigate respondents' beliefs regarding the significance of ovaries versus uteruses. Chapter 2 describes how women who have undergone hysterectomies created a socially constructed hierarchy according to the degree of perceived remaining ovarian function. I expand my analysis of the biological impact of surgery in Chapter 3 by examining the meaning of estrogen replacement therapy for surgically menopausal women.

In Chapters 4, 5, and 6, I describe respondents' post-surgery identity struggles as related to culturally important components of womanhood. These include menstruation in Chapter 4, childbearing in Chapter 5, and sexuality in Chapter 6. Chapter 7 discusses women's endeavors to maintain or reclaim their gender identities through the use of strategies such as *biographical work* and *impression management*. The significance of partners, both male and female, to this process, is also stressed in that chapter.

The variety of answers to the question "Am I still a woman?" are dependent not only on how salient gender identity is for each respondent, but also on her perspective on *what it means to be a woman*. The concluding chapter summarizes my research findings and describes a theory of how gynecological surgery affects gender identity. I close with a discussion of the implications of this research for the identity *woman*.

My goal in this book is to determine the role of gendered body parts in the individual's perception of gender identity. It is intended neither as a self-help book on gynecological surgery nor as a strictly theoretical analysis of gender identity. Through examining the perceptions of hysterectomized women, I hope to shed light not only on their experiences but also on assumptions regarding the necessity of certain body parts for subjective perceptions of women's gender identity. Respondents' discussions of their surgery experiences help problematize the association of organs with gender identity, opening possibilities for re-theorizing essentialist, socialization, and social constructionist theories of sex and gender.

I am firmly committed to the principles of feminist research, including the caveat that this research should be *for* women, rather than simply *on* or *about* women (Reinharz 1992). In addition to theoretical contributions to medical sociology and the sociology of gender, I expect that this book will have practical consequences *for* women who have undergone gynecological surgery, as well as *for* women who may face these surgeries in the future. I have placed women at the center of my study, emphasizing that they are subjects who have agency to resist medical, psychological, and other hegemonic discourses.

2

"Hormonal Hierarchy"

Stratified Stigma Following Hysterectomy

The disciplines of normality, like those of femininity, are not only enforced by others but internalized. For many of us, our proximity to the standards of normality is an important aspect of our identity and our sense of social acceptability, an aspect of our self-respect. We are unlikely to notice this until our ability to meet the standards is threatened in some way.

—*Susan Wendell,* The Rejected Body

The subject at times becomes enmeshed in collusion with forces that sustain her own oppression.

—*Susan Bordo,* Unbearable Weight

Medical Issues Regarding Oophorectomy

The most controversial debate surrounding bilateral salpingo-oophorectomy (bs-o) during hysterectomy involves the removal of healthy ovaries as a prophylaxis for possible future occurrence of ovarian cancer. Fifty-one percent of all hysterectomies performed in the United States involve removal of the ovaries. This includes 40 percent of American women under the age of 45 and 70 percent of older American women who undergo hysterectomy (Lepine et al. 1997). Gynecologists routinely recommend this procedure to women above an arbitrary cut-off age of 40 or 45, with the rationale that they are nearing the age of natural menopause (see Berek 1996, 15, 151). Many of the respondents in my study were considerably younger at the time their ovaries were removed. Although according to the American College of Obstetricians and Gynecologists fewer than 1 percent of women with no history of ovarian tumors and normal-appearing ovaries at the time of hysterectomy will develop cancer in their preserved ovaries (ACOG 1992a) and women who undergo hysterectomy are less likely than other women to develop ovarian cancer (Annegers et al. 1979; Loft, Lindegaard, and Tabor 1997; Parazzini et al. 1993), simply the threat of cancer can frighten women into agreeing to bs-o. However, there can be a sad irony for some women whose healthy ovaries are prophylactically removed. Oncologist Dr. Susan Love cites a medical study published in *Lancet* proving that "contrary to popular belief, you still have some risk of ovarian cancer even if your ovaries are removed. There is ovarian tissue in the areas around the ovary, so that the danger of ovarian cancer, unlike that of uterine cancer, can never be completely eliminated" (1998, 180).

For a premenopausal woman, the loss of hormones resulting from bs-o is thought to create a variety of serious physical problems (BWHBC 1998; Hufnagel 1988; Love 1998). Bs-o instigates "surgical menopause," which differs from natural menopause. Natural menopause is completed over several years, with the last menstrual period occurring for American women at an average age of 51 (ACOG 1992b). While postmenopausal ovaries still continue to produce some estrogens and androgens, bs-o immediately and permanently eliminates this major source of hormone production. Approximately 25 percent of American women reach menopause by way of surgery (Wallis 1995, 51). Of the forty-four total respondents in my study, all of whom had undergone hysterectomies, twenty-seven knew they had also undergone bs-o.[1] Twenty-four of these women were premenopausal prior to bilateral salpingo-oophorectomy. The rationales for respondent's oophorectomies included only benign conditions.

Symbolic Distinctions Between Hysterectomy and Oophorectomy

Decisions regarding oophorectomy are key for many women who undergo hysterectomy. My research indicates that these decisions are not always made due to a strictly medical problem; removal of the ovaries can also involve concerns regarding the construction of female normalcy. While the uterus is most strongly identified with its childbearing function, ovaries are the primary producers of sex hormones, which are popularly considered the essential determinants of sexual difference (Harding 1998; Oudshoorn 1994; Vines 1993). Oophorectomy may therefore carry greater symbolic meaning than hysterectomy, particularly for women who are not interested in bearing (more) children.

Judith Butler (1993) claims that it is important to "name" in order to resignify, recontextualize, and "lay claim" to the meaning of a term. To appropriately "name," it would be proper to refer to women who have undergone bs-o as *castrates*. Although euphemisms such as *oophorectomy, ovariotomy,* or simply *female surgery* may seem less offensive, according to a prominent gynecological text the appropriate medical term for bilateral oophorectomy is "surgical castration" (Berek 1996, 15, 151, 839, 842) since the ovaries are the female gonads, just as the testes are the male gonads. However, despite this medical fact, respondents did not hear their doctors use the term *castration* in reference to their surgeries. This failure to appropriately "name" has left women unprepared to deal with the physical consequences and subjective meanings inherent in the removal of their ovaries that they may discover only *after* surgery.[2]

A number of respondents associated hysterectomy with loss of the ability to bear children but more closely identified oophorectomy with losing something even more essential to their sense of femaleness. Several respondents looked upon hysterectomy as helpful in providing relief from pain or heavy bleeding but felt grief and anger regarding bs-o. This was directly associated with their perceptions of the relative values of uteruses and ovaries with regard to gender identity. For example, Allison, age 27 at the time of surgery, explained that she did not miss her uterus, which she claimed "gave me two good kids but the rest of the time it's been a pain in the butt." However, she told me, "I would probably like some ovaries. I regret that they took those out." Allison made it clear that, while her uterus had "fulfilled its function" by bearing her two children, her ovaries could not "fulfill *their* function of producing female hormones to keep me a woman."

Ethel underw͏ ͏t hysterectomy and bs-o in 1969 at age 46, performed by a surgeon she referred to as "arrogant." She later realized that "maybe they didn't need to take both ovaries; maybe I could have had an ovary left." Ethel still wonders, "Did they need to take *everything*? Because if I had one ovary left, I'd still be making hormones." She was given no explanation as to why both of her ovaries were removed, and during our interview repeatedly returned to discussing her feelings about losing them. Ethel angrily referred to her surgeon as a "typical male chauvinist" who had purposely taken away her "sense of femininity" by unnecessarily removing her ovaries.

Definitions of "Everything"

In describing their surgeries, respondents commonly distinguished between the excision of their uteruses and the removal of *everything*. *Everything* was used as a code word by the majority of respondents. Some of the many examples of their use of this term are as follows:

CATHERINE: *Everything* was completely gone. The cervix, the ovaries, the uterus were completely gone.

INTERVIEWER: How did the doctor explain why he left half an ovary?

PAGE: Because I was too young, he didn't want to take *everything*.

INTERVIEWER: Do you know if they took the ovaries out also? Do you know what they took out?

DOLORES: *Toda.* They took *everything*.

These respondents knew that nothing else had been removed besides their uteruses, ovaries, fallopian tubes, and cervixes. None of them ever mentioned losing a kidney, stomach, urethra, or even an appendix. The all-encompassing term *everything* was used to signify all the internal female sexual/reproductive organs, including the entire uterus, both fallopian tubes, and both ovaries.

Some respondents used *all* as a synonym for *everything*. Sarah's doctor told her she "might just as well take it *all*." Christine asked her surgeon, "Do you have to take *all* the parts out?" He ended-up taking "*everything* except one tenth of one ovary," she reported. Frances explained, "What they did was they took *all* my female parts: my cervix out, *everything* out." Penny was the only respondent who implied more than sexual/reproductive organs in her use of the terms *everything* and *all*; she expanded the meaning of these code words to include other female parts as well. When Penny lost a tremendous amount of weight due to complications of hysterectomy, she lamented, "And I was big-busted and I lost my bust, *everything*. I lost it *all*." She thus extended the meaning to refer to another marker of gender identity—breasts.

Throughout the following discussion regarding ovaries, respondents used the terms *everything* and *all* to indicate the extent of their losses. Most respondents who had undergone bs-o wished that they didn't have to relinquish *everything*. As Yvonne commented after her first surgery: "I had my uterus and cervix taken, but I had my ovaries. It wasn't *everything*." A substantial proportion of respondents who had simple hysterectomies without bs-o expressed relief that they were able to keep their ovaries, which they viewed as necessary to preserve both their femaleness and their femininity. These women discussed femaleness with regard to hormonal balance and sex drive, and femininity in terms of the ability to display appropriate sexual attractiveness. Because respondents did not necessarily have the vocabulary to distinguish between sex and gender, both biological and social meanings are interwoven in their narratives.

Hormonal Hierarchy

Stigma and Gynecological Surgery

Erving Goffman (1963, 2) asserts that "society establishes the means of categorizing persons and the complement of attributes felt to be ordinary and natural for members of each of these categories." He emphasizes that we are not generally aware of our assumptions about the association between certain attributes and social identity until we confront an individual who may not fulfill these assumptions. *Stigma* is produced through the disparity between *virtual* and *actual* social identity. An individual who is different in an important way from other people in his or her social category is "reduced in our minds from a whole and usual person to a tainted, discounted one" (3). According to Goffman, stigma discredits a person, not due to the tainted attribute itself, but because of the "special kind of relationship between attribute and stereotype" (4). For example, individuals considered male are not stigmatized by the absence of uteruses or ovaries, but individuals considered female might be discredited on this basis. A female without a uterus or ovaries might carry a particular type of potential stigma —what Goffman refers to as an "abomination of the body" (5).

Moreover, Goffman maintains, "Stigma involves not so much a set of concrete individuals who can be separated into two piles, the stigmatized and the normal, as a pervasive two-role social process in which every individual participates in both roles. . . . The normal and the stigmatized are not persons but rather perspectives" (1963, 137–38). Individuals who are stigmatized in a particular way may display the same "normal prejudices held toward those who are stigmatized in another regard" (137). Moreover, since the stigmatized individual applies general identity standards to herself, she will inevitably feel ambivalence not only about her own identity but also toward others who are stigmatized in the same way:

> The stigmatized individual exhibits a tendency to stratify his [*sic*]
> 'own' according to the degree to which their stigma is apparent

and obtrusive. He [sic] can then take up in regard to those who are more evidently stigmatized than himself [sic] the attitudes the normals take to him [sic]. Thus do the hard of hearing stoutly see themselves as anything but deaf persons, and those with defective vision, anything but blind. It is in his [sic] affiliation with, or separation from, his [sic] more evidently stigmatized fellows, that the individual's oscillation of identification is most sharply marked. (107)

I noted this inclination of stigmatized individuals to stratify their "own" as a means of identifying with "normals" by distancing themselves from others with related but ostensibly more severe stigmas among respondents with regard to the extent of gynecological surgery. A number of respondents ranked themselves against other women who had undergone hysterectomies, based on whether or not ovaries were removed or on how many ovaries or parts of ovaries had been excised. Some respondents were proud that they kept one or both ovaries, while others expressed remorse that they couldn't retain at least "a piece" of an ovary. These women constructed what I designate as a *hormonal hierarchy*. This hierarchy constitutes what Bury (1982) might refer to as a necessary mobilization of resources to face the crisis in identity initiated by gynecological surgery.

Description of Hormonal Hierarchy

A few respondents were adamant that freedom from annoyance or pain was more important than, as Frances phrased it, "sentimental attachment" to their ovaries. However, the majority of respondents described a form of hierarchy based on the proportion of ovaries they retained following hysterectomy. Respondents whose ovaries were not removed shared the experience of having undergone hysterectomy with women who underwent bs-o; yet, in common with women who have not undergone hysterectomy, they still have ovaries. Significantly, almost every one of these respondents sought to identify with women who had not undergone gynecological surgery. Hanging on to ovaries was a management strategy used to claim membership as part of the in-group including "biologically normal" women and to *disidentify* with the out-group of hysterectomized women who no longer had ovaries (see Sumner 1960). This is not surprising, since other studies have shown that the relationship between social interaction and self-concept is so strong that individuals are unlikely to choose to identify with a stigmatized group (H. M. Strauss 1968). The hormonal hierarchy constructed by respondents assigned the highest value to retaining both ovaries and the lowest value to losing both ovaries. Intermediate values ranged from keeping at least one ovary to saving a tiny piece of an ovary. In general, the goal of women undergoing hysterectomy was to come out of surgery with the best possible approximation of the two-ovary norm. This is connected to the concept that ovaries produce sex hormones, the belief that these sex hormones define womanhood, and the idea that the effects of sex hormones are "qualitatively determined by the quantity of hormones circulating in the blood" (Harding 1998, 58).

Hormonal Hierarchy as a Social Construction

Symbolic interactionist theory asserts that people construct reality based on their cultural experiences. The preceding discussion regarding hormonal hierarchy is founded on respondents' beliefs that different levels of oophorectomy represent *real* distinctions. These beliefs influenced how they viewed their surgeries and compared them to other alternatives and how they compared themselves to other women.

Respondents' constructions of a hormonal hierarchy *may* have a basis in biological fact, but not necessarily, since medical discourse regarding oophorectomy is also socially constructed. A patient education pamphlet distributed by the American College of Obstetricians and Gynecologists continues to advise women: "Even if only one ovary or part of an ovary remains after surgery, it usually will compensate for the loss of the other ovary by producing estrogen and progesterone" (ACOG 1992a). In fact, patient information pamphlets distributed by the ACOG contain contradictory statements regarding ovarian viability following hysterectomy. The patient education pamphlet *The Menopause Years* (ACOG

1992b) states, "While the removal of the uterus alone (hysterectomy) ends periods, it will not cause early menopause. If any part of one or both ovaries remains after surgery, most women will go through menopause around the normal age." Nevertheless, the pamphlet *Understanding Hysterectomy* (ACOG 1992a), published by the same professional medical society, asserts that "[following simple hysterectomy] a woman may go through *menopause* (when menstrual periods end) somewhat sooner than she would have without a hysterectomy. The reasons for this are unclear."

Other medical evidence confirms that even if one or both ovaries remain intact the trauma of hysterectomy alone may interfere with ovarian function (Beavis, Brown, and Smith 1969; Cutler, Garcia, and Edwards 1983; Korenbrot et. al. 1981; Parker et al. 1993; Riedel, Lehmann-Willenbrok, and Semm 1986). Physician Vicki Hufnagel (1989, 25) cites several studies showing that "in more than a third of the cases, the ovaries simply die following a hysterectomy and menopausal symptoms ensue."[3]

Although keeping ovaries was a prize greatly sought by most respondents, the "winners" might be disappointed to find that the hormonal hierarchy does not always have real physiological consequences; the actual value of the retained proportion of a woman's ovaries may be largely symbolic. Nonetheless, when threatened with disruption of their gender identities, most respondents placed great significance on these tiny body parts.[4] For most respondents, the hormonal hierarchy was acted upon as "real in its consequences" (Thomas and Thomas 1927).

Top of the "Hierarchy"

Why do hysterectomized women feel it is important to retain their ovaries? If viewed from a standpoint holding that childbearing is a woman's primary function, it does not make sense to preserve the ovaries. Regardless of the condition of her ovaries, a woman is still unable to bear children after her uterus is removed. This fact may be used to justify a medical decision that remaining ovaries are simply an unnecessary hypothetical source of future pain and disease. Nevertheless, most respondents who retained both ovaries were highly relieved to do so. In addition to the health problems that can be instigated by surgical menopause, these women expressed the symbolic value of knowing that their bodies were still "working" like those of "normal" (i.e., ovulating) women.

The preponderance of respondents placed great significance on keeping both ovaries. Prior to hysterectomy at age 37, Yvonne was relieved to find that she would not undergo oophorectomy simultaneously: "I recall that, when he said that he wouldn't have to take the ovaries, I think I felt that was good. 'This is a bad situation, but at least I'll keep my ovaries.'" Yvonne was forced to return to the hospital twelve years later for a bs-o, but she told me that she was grateful for the time this gave her to experience "natural menopause," which she viewed as a "normal stage for women." Retention of ovaries after her first surgery allowed Yvonne to identify with women who undergo menopause at the appropriate time in their life cycles and to disidentify with women who suffer menopause prematurely or through loss of their ovaries. This is ironic in light of medical evidence that women who retain their ovaries following hysterectomy are more likely to enter menopause earlier than women who have not undergone gynecological surgery (Kaiser, Kusche, and Wurz 1989; Siddle, Sarrel, and Whitehead 1987). Respondents were not generally aware of this possible complication.

Several women initiated conversations with their doctors about keeping their ovaries because they had discussed options with female relatives or friends. Lupe, age 31 at the time of surgery, avoided bs-o through her own persistence, after reading books and magazines and discussing her surgery with a personal medical contact. This respondent believed that she had been literally "burned" by a surgeon who had "screwed-up" a previous tubal ligation by burning the ends of her fallopian tubes rather than simply cutting them so that they could possibly be reattached in the future. By the time she was told she needed a hysterectomy, Lupe, quite understandably, did not trust gynecological surgeons: "I don't know about these doctors. Once they get in there, they just want to take *everything* out." So she took defensive measures. As a receptionist in an internist's office, Lupe spoke to her boss, Dr. Ramirez, about her options. Dr. Ramirez told her that if her ovaries were not affected she should talk to the surgeon about leaving them in so that she wouldn't have to go through surgical menopause at the age of 31. Lupe then warned the surgeon that even if he had to take out her uterus, he had better not remove her ovaries because she "knew there was nothing wrong with them." She put the surgeon on notice that she would check after surgery to ascertain that he didn't take out anything he "wasn't supposed to." Lupe told me that she believed that by preserving her ovaries she would retain her "female hormones and stuff," which she considered crucial to "staying a woman," and which she was not going to "allow him to take them away from [her]."

Joyce, 41 years old at the time of her surgery, understood that her upcoming hysterectomy would provide relief from bleeding benign fibroid cysts. However, she did some informal research that prompted her to interview several gynecologists about the likelihood of removing her ovaries. She selected a particular surgeon because he left the decision up to her. At our interview eight years after surgery, Joyce was still very pleased with her resolution to preserve her ovaries because she strongly considered them a valuable part of her "female body." She believed that it was particularly important to maintain her feminine sex appeal by informing her younger boyfriend that, although she no longer had a uterus, she still had her ovaries, and therefore she "was not going to dry up like a prune." Joyce "felt sorry" for women who did not have the choice to keep their ovaries.

Hormonal "Waxing and Waning"

Yvonne reported that she remained strongly identified as a "normal" woman during the twelve years between hysterectomy and natural menopause: "I just felt that I would still have the same hormonal waxing and waning that I had always had." Although without a uterus Yvonne never again menstruated, she explained, "Well, I would still get sort of premenstrual tension sometimes.

There were times during the month where I would feel more sexual than other times. That kind of thing. So, it was *normal.*"

Joyce described her continued feelings of connection with her hormonal cycle. This persisted although she had not menstruated since her hysterectomy eight years before:

> I still ovulate, because I can feel it. . . . So, um, I—I do think that, um, you know, everything else is basically the same. . . . I—I know that I have a cycle . . . because I know that at certain points of the month, there's still a little mood swing, and I remember that from before. . . . There are certain times of the month, I'll say to myself, 'Why am I feeling this way?' And, um, then, if I know what the date is, I'll say, 'Oooh yes, that's the date!' Um, I kinda know that they're [the ovaries are] still there, and that I haven't gone through menopause. . . . As far as feeling the pain in the middle of the month, sometimes I feel *that* . . . and I don't like any of that, but I guess that makes me aware that, yes, in fact it's still producing estrogen, I—I guess that's what that means . . . if you're ovulating. . . . So, um, I—I guess I'm *glad* about that because I was told that . . . if y-you're not producing estrogen—*your face is gonna dry up* [nervous laugh] and things like that.

Joyce's remaining ovaries clearly allowed her to preserve a sense of female normality, particularly with regard to the "face" she presented to the world.

Like Joyce, Brooke still felt connected to her female hormonal cycle, despite a simple hysterectomy two years earlier. She explained, "I was starting to get the PMS [premenstrual syndrome] again, without having the period." When asked what that was like, Brooke graphically illustrated:

> I still crave chocolates. I still go through major mood changes. I still get very depressed, I still bite people's heads off. . . . I still get some cramping, I still get some pain, but I still have my ovaries. So I'm still ovulating. But it goes to a point and then I just notice that it's gone.

Although Brooke was not entirely happy to have persistent PMS following hysterectomy, she felt that it was worth it to know that her ovaries were working. When I asked her if the PMS feeling was ever so troubling that she wished that her ovaries had been removed, Brooke immediately responded "No," and explained:

> In some ways, *I still identify with other women*. . . . When people sit there and talk about going through PMS, I can still identify, I can still talk about it, *I can still be part of the conversation*. . . . And then they talk about their periods in the same conversation, so I get to say, 'Hah, I don't get mine any more!' That's the beauty of it.

For women like Brooke, preserved ovaries allow them to continue to feel connected to the group of "complete women," despite hysterectomy. Discussing PMS with other women can be seen as a way of managing information to disidentify the stigma of hysterectomy and pass as a "normal" woman (see Goffman 1963).

By contrast, Lupe kept her ovaries but only maintained a connection to her hormonal cycle for a short time. When I asked her how she knew she still had her ovaries after hysterectomy, Lupe told me:

> How do I know they're still there? The other things I'm feeling. You still have times . . . not any more, but the following month I still felt that I had that kind of function in me [ovulation in the middle of the month]. And when I was feeling it, I would consult and they would tell me, 'Well it's just your ovaries; they have their function. They have to get used to working without the uterus.' . . . I felt the pain the first month after, that I would feel just before the period. But then right after that it was gone.

Lupe sounded wistful that she no longer had this physical sign of her hormonal cycle. She lamented, "I know women who still get bloating sometimes. They bloat even without having the uterus, but they have their ovaries. I don't even get that. It's like I got rid of *everything*." Lupe envied other women who continued to experience physical signs that their ovaries were still active. These physical signs indicate that women are at the top of the hormonal hierarchy. Absence of these markers leaves doubt. It is ironic that, in order to affirm their status as women, respondents appropriated symptoms of premenstrual syndrome (PMS) and premenstrual tension (PMT), usually perceived as problematic, to affirm their status as "women."

"In the land of the blind, the one-eyed man is king": Unilateral Oophorectomy

If those women who retained both ovaries are at the top of the hormonal hierarchy, placed somewhat lower are those women who managed to keep one ovary. Since some medical advice indicates that as long as a woman retains one ovary, or even a piece of an ovary, she is capable of producing all her "female hormones," most respondents were relieved to keep whatever remnant they could. Prior to her hysterectomy, Anita was told that "if they could save the ovaries, they would, but if not, then *everything* would have to go." Afterward, she was informed that "I had one ovary that was good, the other one was bad. So he [the surgeon] just took it out. I have my right ovary, but the left was bad."

Several other women talked in terms of "bad ovaries" that were useless, or (even worse) pernicious, and "good ovaries" that were worth saving. At the time of her hysterectomy, her surgeon told Gloria, age 39, that she couldn't be certain about whether she would have to remove her ovaries until she was "in there." Post-surgery, Gloria was pleased to find that only one ovary had been removed. She explained that, since she was premenopausal, the ovary was left "to let it do its work" of keeping her "a functioning female."

Leave Me a Little Piece

If they could not keep at least one "good ovary," some respondents were gratified that they were still able to preserve a "good piece of an ovary." Theoretically, even a small amount of remaining ovarian tissue can continue to produce sufficient estrogen, thus placing these women higher on the hormonal hierarchy than those who had undergone bs-o. Page told me that after her hysterectomy at age 33, "[The doctor] left a little piece of an ovary, hoping it would take over and provide me with the hormones that I needed, which it did do." Although it had to be removed seven years later, Page is convinced that keeping that portion of ovary "worked out very, very well." When I asked Page to clarify in what way this piece of ovary "worked well," she explained that her ovarian hormones continued to function, allowing her to preserve "my sense of femininity."

According to Christine, who was 38 at the time of her hysterectomy for benign fibroid tumors and endometriosis, the surgeon removed "*everything* except one-tenth of one ovary." When I asked her why he had left that piece of ovary, she explained:

> He left the only thing he thought was still healthy. . . . So that I would still have some estrogen production. And it worked. Not immediately. What he didn't tell me, but I had read it, so I knew. It shuts down temporarily and then you have to hope it kicks in again, and mine did [two months later].

Christine believes that the tiny remaining piece of ovary enabled her to produce her own estrogen, the quintessential female hormone, for another seven years. She reported that she "felt sorry" for those women who "lost all their ovaries, and have no female hormones left."

Later Regrets

Respondents who regretted losing their ovaries most bitterly were those women who had agreed to bs-o prior to their hysterectomies but reconsidered their decisions after their surgeries when it was too late. Isabella, whose native language is Spanish, said, "They told me they had to take one ovary because I have a problem, but the other is good. But in the future, they have to take it out. It's better do it now and not wait a couple of years." Frightened by the prospect of future surgery, although not fully comprehending other possibilities, Isabella agreed to bs-o, a decision she now laments. Although she knew she would never have had more children due to a previous tubal ligation, Isabella, 39, told me that she still grieved over the loss of her "woman parts."

Alice actually initiated the idea of bs-o with her surgeon, much to her later regret. Upon finding that she needed a hysterectomy due to hemorrhaging fibroids, she considered it fortunate that she could consult her sister-in-law, who is a gynecologist. Alice explained:

> And she [the sister-in-law] said to me, she was the one who said to me, "Alice, you're 43, or something like that, those organs can only get into more trouble as you get older. . . ." And I said I didn't want to have any more problems. So she suggested that I suggest to the doctors that I didn't mind if they took *everything*. . . . But I really didn't understand until after it was done, what it meant. . . . I had no idea. I really didn't understand what happened to your body once they took *everything*. I had no idea. I had no idea—I didn't understand it.

Alice later came to feel that she had needed the hysterectomy but had made a grave mistake regarding the removal of her ovaries. She greatly missed experiencing the female hormonal cycle to which she had been accustomed. "I was faced with nothing to regulate whatever psychological thing I had always done for so many years," Alice told me. "I was angry at myself for not understanding this powerful thing that would happen to my body." She was also furious with her gynecologist sister-in-law, to whom she no longer speaks. Although the loss of her ovaries was emotionally devastating, Alice was unable to share her feelings with anyone: "It was my own private shock." She didn't feel entitled to complain, "because I had already made the decision and I had to live with this now." Like Isabella, Alice's emotional pain was exacerbated by her belief that she had signed the death warrant for her own ovaries, which she saw in retrospect as valued parts of her "womanhood."

Thus, gynecological surgery prompts women to consider the meanings of their wombs and ovaries, generally taken for granted as "natural" components of female bodies. Respondents' experiences indicate that the ovaries may carry greater symbolic meaning regarding gender identity than does the uterus. While the uterus is strongly identified with its childbearing function, ovaries, which are the female gonads, are known to produce sex hormones, popularly believed to be the essence of sex difference. Respondents translated their understandings that womanhood is created and maintained by the existence of specific hormones into an elaborate hormonal hierarchy. This hierarchy is a social construction whereby respondents who had undergone hysterectomy ranked themselves according to how close they measure up to the two-ovary norm following surgery.

In describing their surgeries, respondents commonly distinguished between excision of their uteruses and the removal of *everything*. Several women believed that they were able to maintain a connection to their former physical female selves because retained ovaries (or parts of ovaries) following hysterectomy allowed their "female" hormones to continue cycling, despite the fact that without uteruses they no longer experienced menstrual bleeding. While this may be debatable as medical fact, respondents who retained both ovaries, one ovary, or even a portion of an ovary were less likely to question their gender normalcy following hysterectomy. Thus, bs-o may instigate greater biographical disruption of gender identity than does hysterectomy alone. As demonstrated by my analysis of respondents' perceptions, this phenomenon may be created both through tangible hormonal effects and through the social construction of gendered biology. The hormonal hierarchy represents more than differences among women in their sense of loss—it describes status designations. Identity as a woman was highly valued by nearly all respondents, and they sought to preserve this normative status.

3

An "Ovary Prosthesis"?

The Meanings of Estrogen Replacement Therapy

There is widespread belief in our society that drugs create dependence and that being on chemical substances is not a good thing. Somehow, whatever the goal is, it is thought to be better if we can get there without drugs.

—*Peter Conrad, "The Meaning of Medications"*

MENOPAUSE IS not always a "midlife" event; as many as 25 percent of American women reach it by way of surgery. Natural menopause is completed over several years, with the last period occurring at an average age of 51 for American women (ACOG 1992a,b). In contrast, surgical removal of both ovaries instigates immediate and sudden "surgical menopause." Furthermore, while the ovaries of naturally menopausal women continue to produce some hormones for the remainder of their lives, women who undergo bilateral salpingo-oophorectomy (bs-o), or whose ovaries cease functioning due to hysterectomy, lose this primary source of estrogens and androgens.[1] For premenopausal women, the abrupt loss of ovarian hormones may cause a variety of serious physical problems, including possible greater susceptibility to heart disease, osteoporosis, arthritis, chronic illness, benign breast disease, joint pain and immobility, chronic fatigue, and urinary incontinence as well as short-term memory loss and increased levels of depression, mood disorders, and neurological diseases. Additional problems may include vaginal dryness and thinning, excessively dry skin, vasomotor symptoms (including "hot flashes" and "night sweats"), proliferation of body hair, and greater reliance upon prescription drugs.[2] This chapter explores the meanings women have assigned to estrogen replacement therapy, which is commonly prescribed for women who have undergone surgical menopause.

Estrogen replacement therapy (ERT) refers to the administration of an exogenous form of estrogen in order to raise estrogen levels. Hormone replacement therapy (HRT) is a broader term that commonly refers to a combination of exogenous estrogen and progesterone (or progestin). There is a common confusion regarding the distinctions between these types of hormone replacement therapy. While estrogen replacement therapy alone (ERT) is generally administered to women who have undergone hysterectomies, only combined therapy (HRT) is administered to women who retain their uteruses. The reason for these different hormone therapies is that ERT alone was found to cause cancer of the uterine lining, obviously not a problem for hysterectomized women. Although several sociologists (e.g., Bell 1987; Grossman and Bart 1979; Kaufert 1982; Kaufert and McKinlay 1985; Koeske 1982; McCrea 1983) have studied HRT in connection with natural menopause, there is a dearth of sociological studies about women's experiences with ERT for surgical menopause.

Twenty-six respondents knew that they had undergone bilateral salpingo-oophorectomies (bs-o). Their ages ranged from 27 to 69 years old at the time of surgery, with an average age of 41.4 and a median age of 40. Twenty-four of these women were premenopausal prior to bs-o and thus experienced surgical menopause. Of the twenty-four respondents who underwent surgical menopause, all but one had been on ERT at some point, and twenty were currently taking ERT at the time of their interviews.

As discussed in the previous chapter, estrogen is popularly seen as the quintessential "female hormone" despite the fact that men also produce estrogen (Harding 1998; Oudshoorn 1994; Vines

1993). Women were very aware of their positions in the hormonal hierarchy because they perceived that femaleness and femininity were produced and maintained by sufficient levels of estrogen. Therefore, many respondents viewed their lack of ovaries as a gender disability and believed that ERT acted as a kind of "ovary prosthesis."

Medicalization vs. Medical Treatment for Medically Induced Problems

Medicalization of Natural Menopause

"Medicalization" is the process by which the social control of medicine is extended over areas of life that were previously considered nonmedical (Freidson 1970; Schneider and Conrad 1980; Zola 1972). Medical sociologists have noted that women's life stages, including menstruation, childbirth, and menopause, are particularly prone to medicalization (see Conrad 1992; Riessman 1989). Oudshoorn (1994) indicates that hormone manufacturers focused on marketing hormone therapy to women because they were more accessible as patients than men, for whom there is no equivalent to gynecologists.

One brand of ERT, Premarin, was the most prescribed of all drugs in the United States for many years and only recently has dropped to third. More than 45 million prescriptions for Premarin were dispensed in 2001, for a total of $2.75 billion spent on all hormone therapy in that year (Grady 2002a). HRT and ERT are generally administered as pills, but many women take exogenous hormones in the form of skin patches, topical cream, or subdermal injection. Newer treatments include vaginal suppositories and implants. At the time of respondents' interviews, I found that both medical authorities and women's health activists generally discussed taking hormones as a matter of "personal choice." However, while medical sources minimized potential risks, women's health activists were skeptical of potential benefits.[3] As a result of the more recent findings from large-scale research studies on hormone therapy, both medical sources and the popular media have begun to view hormone therapy with the same alarm as do women's health activists.

By defining menopause as a "natural" physiological event that has been medicalized, women's health activists have performed an important public service. They have contested previous cultural constructs of menopausal women as "no longer functional women," "past their prime," "castrates," or "unsexed" (see Coney 1994; Corea 1977; Fausto-Sterling 1985; Voda 1997). Spearheaded by the Boston Women's Health Book Collective and the National Women's Health Network, both academic (e.g., Callahan 1993; Komesaroff, Rothfield, and Daly 1997) and popular books (e.g., Greer 1992; LeGuin 1976; Sheehy 1992) aimed at midlife women focus on the positive side of menopause—less responsibility for childrearing, new opportunities for self-expression, and a "menopausal zest."[4] The women's health movement has even had an impact on the medical profession's public discussion of menopause. In a patient information pamphlet available in gynecologists' offices, the American College of Obstetricians and Gynecologists officially states:

> There are a lot of myths about menopause—the time in a woman's life when she stops menstruating. It s a normal stage of life, as natural as pregnancy or menstruation. . . . Many good years lie ahead after menopause. The physical changes that occur during menopause should not prevent you from enjoying this time of life. (ACOG 1992b)

However, despite this growing recognition that natural menopause is a normal life stage, medical authorities continue to refer to combined hormone therapy as hormone *replacement* therapy, implying that naturally menopausal women have lost something that needs to be replaced.[5] Women's health advocates argue against the accuracy of this terminology.

Feminist sociological research during the 1970s and 1980s demonstrated that the development of hormone therapy was instrumental in the medicalization of natural menopause. The following statement by Susan Bell is characteristic: "They [medical specialists] transformed the meaning of menopause and defined it as a medical problem with a medical solution; they labeled it a 'deficiency disease'" (1987, 539). According to McCrea, leaders of the women's health movement implicated the use of ERT as "exploitation and an insidious form of social control" (1983, 111).

Recent feminist research continues to make the case against hormone therapy for the treatment of natural menopause (Callahan 1993; Gonyea 1996; Harding 1997; Klein and Dumble 1994; Lewis 1993; Oakley 1998; Worcester and Whatley 1992). Even before more conclusive medical findings regarding the negative effects of HRT, many popular books and newsletters written by women's health activists encouraged women to resist the medicalization of natural menopause.[6] There is some evidence that general cultural attitudes toward menopause have improved in the past thirty years (Weinstein 1997). However, for the 25 percent of American women who undergo bs-o premenopausally, including twenty-six respondents in my study, menopause is not an expected life stage event or a "natural unfolding." For these women, surgical menopause is a medically induced event that is not "normal."

Medically Induced Problems

Unfortunately, the appropriate emphasis on menopause as a "normal" stage of life may in fact heighten the stigma of surgical menopause. Several respondents remarked that they felt excluded from menopause self-help literature whose general message is that all women who "live long enough" will go through the predictable stage of natural menopause. Ironically, this reinforced for them the concept that menopause at midlife is "normal" and that they were therefore "abnormal" because they were chronologically out of sync. Taking prescription medication for a medical condition thus carried different meanings for respondents who underwent surgical menopause than it might for women passing through a normal stage of life. For example, Kelly, a nurse practitioner who had undergone hysterectomy and bs-o at 45, said she was grateful that ERT was available to her. "I think I need it," she told me. "I think I had traumatic surgery. And I'm relatively young compared to most women who go through menopause, and I can see the risks."

Women's health activists have generally focused critiques of hormone therapy on the medical and pharmaceutical establishments rather than on individual women. In addition, although strongly opposed to HRT for naturally menopausal women, several women's health activists now acknowledge the effectiveness of ERT for surgically menopausal women:

> We support the use of estrogen by women whose ovaries are removed before age forty-five. In this context, ERT is truly "replacement" therapy, although we emphasize that no pill can replace all of the various hormones lost by surgical removal of the ovaries, nor mimic accurately the delicate interaction among several hormones. (NWHN 2002, 42)

Despite this, the common conflation in popular media regarding HRT for natural menopause and ERT for surgical menopause prompted some respondents to feel defensive about their decisions to take ERT. Christine told me that, after her sister had a hysterectomy and bs-o at age 28, "she decided not to take estrogen, based on what we read from the women's community." This sister suffered horrible pain as the result of vaginal atrophy and became deeply depressed as a result. Christine commented that she thought her sister "made a foolish decision [to refrain from taking ERT], but then I understood the conflicts she felt." Following her own surgery at age 38, Christine decided that she would take ERT, even though she believed that this was contradictory to the position of some "women's health activists who warned against it." In addition to pharmaceutical advertisements proclaiming that hormone therapy was a wonder drug, several other respondents perceived a competing discourse in some self-help books. This alternate discourse implied that taking hormone therapy constituted a misguided weakness, and they therefore felt that it was necessary for them to defend their decisions to take ERT.

A number of respondents attempted to avoid taking hormone medication but later were resigned to recognizing that their situations were significantly different than that of naturally menopausal women. Margie, a nurse who underwent bs-o at 33, explained:

> I had read a lot. I think I was going to wait and see what happened and then make the decision [regarding ERT], but I felt like a French fry in the recovery room. . . . I was like hot as hell. I personally feel like I need it.

Like most respondents in her position, Margie did not believe that drug companies had pushed hormone therapy on her; she was gratified to find a medical cure for a medically induced problem.[7] In view of my finding that the vast majority of respondents felt empowered by their decisions to take ERT, it is interesting to note that, even prior to the more recent negative announcements regarding HRT, hormone therapy compliance rates were generally much higher for women who experienced surgical menopause than for those who underwent natural menopause (Cauley et al. 1990; Hemminki et al. 1991; Johannes et al. 1994). Although hormone therapy has been very widely prescribed to American women, many naturally menopausal women have never filled their hormone prescriptions. Thus, for reasons that were clarified by respondents in my study, both hysterectomy and youth are significantly associated with hormone use (Finley et al. 2001).

That reactions to medical prescriptions differ between women who experience menopause as part of the life course and those who undergo a medical event seems reasonable. Respondents commonly referred to ERT as a strategy to recover control of their female body chemistry and to retain or regain youth and femininity. At first glance, these rationales appear very similar to those often offered by naturally menopausal women for taking HRT. However, a more thorough analysis reveals that there are important differences both in material circumstances and in symbolic meanings for these two groups of women.

Gender-Related Rationales for Taking Estrogen Replacement Therapy

ERT as a Strategy to Recover Control of the Hormonal Body

A *hormonal body* is a body that is perceived as being controlled by hormones, according to Jennifer Harding (1998). Several other researchers confirm that hormones are widely viewed as mechanisms of bodily control and that the female body is seen as particularly controlled by hormones (e.g., Oodshoorn 1994; Vines 1993). A key theme throughout the narratives of surgically menopausal respondents was the experience of losing control of bodily function through medical intervention. For example, Alice told me that, prior to surgery, "I felt that I could control my body." However, the severe vasomotor symptoms that began immediately following hysterectomy and bs-o made her feel "out of control." "The hot flashes were such a shock!" she exclaimed. "I had no clue that this would happen. . . . I had always been so in charge!" At first Alice fought medical recommendations to take ERT because she wanted to "handle this" herself, but she finally succumbed, believing that she needed medication to help her "regulate" her body. "I realized I *had* to take this Premarin," she declared. "If I missed this pill by even an hour, all of a sudden I was like drenched [as the result of sweating due to hormone withdrawal]!" A number of respondents complained that, like Alice, they felt like they had "lost control" of their own bodies following surgical removal of their ovaries. Arguably, this was partly the result of the medical invasion of their bodies through surgery, but respondents mentioned this rationale less often than they discussed the loss of control they felt due to missing "female hormones."[8]

Women who undergo surgical menopause are younger (sometimes by decades) than women who experience natural menopause. In addition, the vasomotor symptoms of surgical menopause are generally much more sudden, frequent, and physically devastating (Berek 1996; Rock and Thompson 1997). These vasomotor symptoms include "hot flashes" and "night sweats," both of which can significantly affect quality of life. In addition, these symptoms can be very obvious to other people, making highly visible the otherwise invisible stigma of premature menopause and "spoiling identity" (Goffman 1963). Many respondents viewed ERT as a way of gaining control not only of their medical symptoms but also of premature menopause itself. For instance, Madison, age 39 at surgery, claimed that ERT allowed her to be "more in charge": "I'm glad I didn't have to go through menopause yet," she told me, "It's sort of gonna be within my control, I guess."

ERT to Secure Youth and Femininity

STAYING YOUNG. As discussed in the previous chapter, estrogen is widely viewed as the quintessential "female sex hormone"—the primary determiner that makes a woman a woman. Respondents indicated that ERT not only relieved severe physical consequences of surgical menopause, but replacing estrogen (viewed as "the female hormone") had great symbolic gender value for them as well. In popular American culture, youth and beauty are crucial requirements for public confirmation of femininity, and beginning in the 1960s, estrogen therapy was "promoted by physicians and the pharmaceutical industry as a way of avoiding menopause and preserving youth and beauty" (McCrea 1983, 111). Women's health activists often cite a formerly popular book by a noted medical authority claiming that ERT can "turn back the clock." McCrea argues that menopausal women "are vulnerable to the promise of a 'youth' pill which purports to allay the aging process" (1983, 120). More recently, Lock claims, "A potent fear of aging, coupled with a quest for immortal youthfulness and sexual desire, seems to be driving the medicalization of menopause" (1993, 367).

However, respondents who mentioned ERT as a strategy to delay menopause did not imply that they were attempting to achieve "eternal youth"; they asserted that they merely wanted the opportunity to experience youth while they were still young. As Susan declared, "I just didn't want to be sixty when I was only fifty!" Sunny stated that she decided to take ERT following bilateral oophorectomy at age 41 because "I just didn't feel like I was ready to go through menopause. My thought, exactly, was, "I'm not ready to prune up." Although women who undergo natural menopause may also be reluctant to "prune up," there is a difference between yearning to be younger and simply wanting to seem the "correct" biological age.

Several sociologists have examined the importance of biographical timing in relation to chronic illness. According to Gubrium, Holstein, and Buckholdt, "Notions of a typical life course . . . serve as an interpretive resource for discerning normality in relation to chronological age. The image of being 'on time' or 'off time' often leads to attributions of normality or accusations of deviance, abnormality, or deficiency" (1994, 79; see also Zerubavel 1981). Others have studied the phenomenon of being "off time" for young adults living with arthritis (Bury 1982) and Parkinson's disease (Singer 1974). They find that a condition implying premature aging marks "a biographical shift from a perceived normal trajectory through relatively chronological steps, to one fundamentally abnormal and inwardly damaging" (Bury 1982, 171).

With specific regard to menopause, an analysis of data from a survey conducted by the National Center for Health Statistics concludes: "When menopause occurs on time, i.e., during midlife, it is not associated with psychological distress. When menopause occurs at earlier or later stages of the life course, however, psychological distress may ensue" (Lennon 1982, 353).[9] Other researchers (McKinlay, McKinlay, and Brambilla 1987) have found that women who had undergone surgical menopause were much more likely to experience depression than were women who underwent or anticipated natural menopause. For many oophorectomized respondents, taking ERT was a means to prevent the symptoms of premature menopause, thus theoretically enabling them to maintain their chronological age status as young women.

RETAINING OR REGAINING FEMININITY.   A number of respondents believed that ERT was an effective replacement for missing ovaries and the "female" hormones they produce. Most striking is the experience of Catherine, age 32 at the time of surgical menopause, who began ERT in her late sixties after approximately thirty years without it. When speaking about this, Catherine declared, "Hooray! I'm a woman again!" I asked what that meant, and she explained, "Well, my breasts were like dragging and sagging, and they became fuller. I felt my whole body change." Catherine summed up her beliefs regarding the relationship of ERT to her gender identity as follows:

> I just felt like a female again. I mean, I always felt like a female, but for a long time without that, without really thinking about it . . . it's a strange thing. What happens is, when your body changes like that, when the hormones are off, you keep going, but you don't— *you don't really feel like a woman.*

Kelly, a nurse who became surgically menopausal at age 45, strongly connected her femininity with "female" hormones. "I think we're very hormonal," she told me. "I think women have a lot more hormonal effect on our thinking, our sensitivity, and stuff. It really has to do with our hormone fluxes." She connected estrogen to the female ability to express emotion: "Yeah, well they talk—I've had men who are very sensitive and they say, 'Gee, he must have more estrogen in his body!'" She implied that this was the converse of a woman who has too little estrogen.[10]

After Allison's bs-o at age 28, she felt "altered" and first went to a male gynecologist who was adamant that she didn't need hormone therapy because, as she put it, "it was all in my head." She switched to a female gynecologist who helped her experiment with different dosage levels of ERT. Allison believed that she needed replacement estrogen "due to the fact that I don't have my own chemicals that my body produces." We had the following exchange:

ALLISON: I thought I was going to grow a penis if they didn't do something! I mean I was really . . .

INTERVIEWER: Why do you say that?

ALLISON: My husband and I have a joke about that—if I don't take my estrogen, I'm going to grow a penis. . . .

INTERVIEWER: How do you mean that? That you were going to grow a penis?

ALLISON: Well, I just think that your body becomes not yourself.

INTERVIEWER: In what way?

ALLISON: Emotionally, physically . . .

As a former medical technician, Allison obviously did not literally believe that she would grow a penis or turn into a man if she didn't take ERT. However, she did perceive that estrogen deprivation made her feel less womanly. At the time of her interview, Allison had taken ERT for thirteen years and had no intention of stopping. Although, like most respondents, securing gender identity was not the only reason she took ERT, it was an important underlying theme in her choice to do so.

Some respondents were surprised that ERT failed to preserve all aspects of their femininity. Isabella actually stopped taking Premarin because she was disappointed that it had an adverse effect on the cultural ideal that women are supposed to be slender: "Ummm, I'm afraid to take them because I find out my weight was coming higher. . . . It is very difficult to lose weight when you are taking the pills." While ERT may have been a ticket to feeling more "womanly" for some women, it did not provide a passport to the embodiment of limitless femininity.

Respondents disagreed as to which brand of ERT provided the most "normal" type of estrogen. Premarin, the most widely prescribed form, is advertised as derived from "natural" sources.[11] Nevertheless, Premarin may be natural only if the female taking it has four legs and eats hay, since it is synthesized from the urine of pregnant mares. It is also debatable whether estrogens like Estrace, Estratab, or Ogen, which are manufactured from other sources, are exactly the same as estrogens found naturally in premenopausal women. Despite the popular movement among menopausal baby boomers to "go natural" by using plant estrogens (phytoestrogens) rather than those developed in laboratories (Shandler 1997), only a couple of respondents had considered this option. This is probably due to the very unnatural circumstance of surgical menopause.[12]

A few respondents chose to go beyond ERT in seeking to achieve a hormonal balance as close as possible to that of a "normal" premenopausal woman. To this end, they decided to take combined HRT, including progesterone (progestin) as well as estrogen. One respondent, Andrea, age 36 at surgery, even insisted that her gynecologist prescribe combined therapy with testosterone because she believed that this form of HRT would reproduce a more "normal" female hormone equilibrium: "My body had produced that, and the fact that it wasn't being put in my body meant that something was out of balance." Andrea found that her male gynecologist was very reluctant to prescribe testosterone, which is usually considered a "male" hormone. She attributed her doctor's aversion to sexism.

Previous research indicates that taking medication can reinforce feelings of stigma in sufferers (Conrad 1985). I found that ERT did sometimes remind women of the potential stigma of missing ovaries. Respondents disagreed as to whether taking exogenous estrogen in either pill or patch forms made them feel more "normal," although the majority took oral estrogen. Following bilateral oophorectomy at age 39, Janet felt that taking a daily Premarin pill was depressing because it reminded her that she *had* to take it due to absent ovaries. However, she did not want to switch to an estrogen patch because she thought it might be a constant externally visible reminder to herself and her partner. She suggested a preferable alternative: "It would be great to hear that they've found a way to transplant ovaries, or even implant artificial ones."[13]

"Resisters," "Stoics," and "Martyrs": The Decision Not to Take Hormones

Only one respondent who had undergone surgical menopause had never taken any form of ERT, and twenty were still taking it at the time of their interviews. For a couple of women, exogenous estrogen was contraindicated by their present medical conditions. For example, Page took ERT after hysterectomy at age 33 and bs-o at age 40. "I loved it," she said. Unfortunately, her doctors insisted she stop taking ERT because she had developed skin melanomas. Barbara was taken off Premarin very soon after surgery because she developed blood clots in her legs. At our interview two months later, she was unsure whether her doctor would allow her to take ERT since estrogen was implicated as possible origin of this disorder. Barbara told me that she hoped that she would be allowed to resume ERT in order to "restore lost hormones."

Frances was the only respondent who was adamant about *not* taking ERT. She had discussed exogenous hormones with her gynecologist but decided, "I really have no thought that I'm ever going to need that. I don't think I'm ever going to have any menopause symptoms. I feel great." However, it is important to point out that Frances was 49 at the time of surgery, considerably older than most surgically menopausal respondents. She was well within the age range for natural menopause and may have already begun the gradual lowering of hormone levels that occurs during the perimenopause at the time of her surgery.

Most respondents maintained that every woman should decide for herself whether or not to take exogenous hormones. However, rather than glorifying women who resisted hormone therapy, as is often done by women's health activists, several respondents stated that they thought a refusal to take ERT was "absurd." Some believed that women who declined ERT in order to "tough it out" were expressing a negative kind of "he-man attitude." Allison was one respondent who negatively characterized women who rejected ERT: "I've seen women deciding that they are going to be really stoic and not go with estrogen, and, God, some of them. . . . I've seen women who are trying to do without it, and they are just miserable, and it's like, God. . . . Forget it, this is *ridiculous!*"

Ann, a feminist health educator who had previously argued against the use of hormone therapy, told me that she had no desire to be "a martyr." Post-surgery, she had "only one middle-of-the-night experience that was so huge I didn't even realize what it was." Her female partner suggested that maybe it was a hot flash.

"It was horrible! So I didn't ever want to have another one," Ann stated. She said she was feeling great and saw no reason to stop taking ERT, despite what she perceived was the "politically correct" attitude of *not* taking hormones: "I teach a course on women and health and I have to listen to people going on and on. And I just listen quietly. I have these 20-year-olds; they write these muckraking essays about the American medical establishment, blah, blah, blah. It's really stupid." Thus, several respondents inverted the cultural concept (Conrad 1985, 156–57) that avoiding medication is a virtue.

"Catch-22": Possible Long-term Benefits and Risks of ERT

Medical Control and Medical Uncertainty

Most respondents were well aware of controversies regarding long-term health effects of hormone therapy. Possible benefits and risks are not only discussed in gynecological texts and medical journals,[14] but also in patient education pamphlets in doctors' offices,[15] and popular books written by both doctors and women's health activists.[16] Popular newspapers and magazines also frequently run articles on the prospects and perils of hormone therapy. According to these various sources, ERT may carry several long-term health benefits, including prevention of osteoporosis, lowering LDL ("bad") cholesterol levels and raising HDL ("good") cholesterol levels, strengthening blood vessels, and relief or prevention of bladder and urinary problems and vaginal atrophy. There is considerable debate over whether ERT also decreases the risk of fatal heart disease, delays skin aging, relieves depression or other psychological symptoms, or increases sexual desire. Unfortunately, ERT may also carry a number of risks—some merely bothersome, others quite dangerous. The less severe consequences may include breast tenderness, leg cramps, fluid retention, bloating, migraine headaches, weight gain, nausea, and vaginal discharge. More dangerous possible consequences are greater risk of breast cancer and gallstones, recurrence of endometriosis and fibroids, and increased potential for stroke and heart disease.

While a number of researchers warn women about "the consequences of passively accepting whatever they were told by their physicians" (Kaufert and McKinlay 1985, 133), others document that individuals do not necessarily take medications in passive compliance of medical authority (Conrad 1985; 1987a; Peyrot, McMurray, and Hedges 1987; Schneider and Conrad 1983). I found that most respondents in my study were not passive with regard to medical advice regarding hormone therapy. Regardless of educational or class level, women used a variety of methods to determine whether to take ERT, including reading self-help manuals, magazine articles, and information published by women's health activists; medical and social science research; and, most frequently, discussions with mothers, sisters, friends, and other female relatives and acquaintances. Having conducted some research, many of these respondents believed that they were making independent and rational decisions regarding ERT.

One of these women was Sunny, age 41 at the time of her hysterectomy and bs-o, who told me that that she felt that the choice of whether to take ERT was up to her. She said that her doctor told her "exactly what would happen to my body if I took it and exactly what would happen if I didn't take it, and asked me what I wanted to do." Sunny believed she had made an intelligently informed choice and was not coerced into taking medication. However, medical uncertainty makes it impossible to determine "exactly" what consequences she, or any woman, might face as a result of ERT. For example, even though Sunny was confident that she was not at risk for breast cancer because there was no history of breast cancer in her family, less than 10 percent of breast cancers actually stem from inherited causes (Massachusetts Breast Cancer Coalition 1996), and the medical data are mixed with regard to the effects of ERT on future breast cancer. Although Sunny believed that she was making a reasoned decision, there is actually no conclusive way to determine hypothetical risks and benefits without the advice of a clairvoyant.

A number of respondents complained that they were bewildered by the ambiguous advice they were given regarding ERT. In this regard, medical uncertainty was a much more crucial problem than was medical control. Lyons and Griffin find that menopause is represented in self-help texts as a time when women are charged with making "sensible and responsible decisions regarding their health and future well-being," and that "taking hormone therapy is discussed as a sensible and responsible choice if there are no major medical contraindications" (2000, 473). However, several women complained to me that it is irrational to make a rationale choice based on uncertainty. They bitterly described the conflicting messages regarding ERT that they have tried to cope with over the years.

Ethel's story is not atypical of the dilemma women faced when they attempted to be well informed regarding ERT choices. In 1969, following her hysterectomy and bs-o at the age of 46, Ethel's gynecologist informed her that she had to take Premarin, while her internist insisted that estrogen was dangerous due to unknown health risks. He said he would rather prescribe a mild sleeping pill for her terrible night sweats. Several months later, Ethel felt much better and thought, "Why take medication that you don't need?" So she decided not to take ERT. Unfortunately, a number of years later Ethel had a very severe back problem and was told by the orthopedic surgeon, "You *must* be on hormones. Your back is too thin . . . your bones are so thin, your back bone density is so thin—when you fall, we're going to have to get a shovel and dustpan and sweep up all the pieces!" At this point, Ethel went on ERT for about two years. But then, she told me, "I kept reading these articles about the increased risk of breast cancer with the hormones. And I took myself off, and I didn't go back on them until we moved here."[17]

Sixteen years after she stopped ERT, Ethel started taking Premarin again, although she said she felt "fairly well" while off it. She explained, "My son, in the meantime, went to medical school, and he has always been after me to be on hormones." A bone density test showed mild osteoporosis in her wrist, and her son advised,

"Mom, you should be on Premarin." He told her there are risks with everything but, he said, "I think in your case, there are also other benefits." Ethel, although a very smart woman, was still confused. She told me, "My internist here . . . in their office, there are four doctors there. Two of them are for Premarin hormones, and two are against, right in the same office!"

As was the case for other respondents, Ethel not only got conflicting advice regarding whether she should take ERT, but her physicians could not even agree what regimen she should follow if she did take estrogen. When she resumed taking ERT, her internist cautioned her to take it for only twenty-one days per month.[18] However, when Ethel had surgery for a bladder prolapse in 1989, the gynecologist informed her that "since I had a total hysterectomy, he would like to see me take Premarin every day of my life. . . . He said, 'Why stop at twenty-one [days]? You *need* it!'" No wonder even intelligent, well-read women can feel like human Ping-Pong balls, bouncing between different perspectives on ERT. Rather than protesting that they are dominated by medical control, respondents complained that choices regarding ERT are in their hands but that the conflicting options are overwhelming. The results of more recent research regarding hormone therapy only make this issue more confusing for women who have undergone hysterectomy and bs-o.

Recent Research Regarding HRT and the Implications for ERT

As I described earlier in this chapter, many women's health activists have long argued against the safety and efficacy of HRT and have campaigned for large-scale, randomized, controlled clinical trials to determine actual risks and benefits to menopausal women. In 1998 the results of the Heart and Estrogen/Progestin Replacement Study (HERS) became available. This study included 2,763 participants, all of whom had been previously diagnosed with heart disease and who had intact uteruses. The HERS trial found that taking HRT for up to four years did not prevent further heart attacks or death from previous heart disease despite a positive influence on cholesterol levels. In fact, this study found an elevated risk for coronary heart disease during the first year of hormone therapy (Grady, Herrington, and Bittner et al. 2002). In 2001 the American Heart Association cautioned that women should not consider hormone replacement as a means to either treat or prevent heart disease (Grady 2002a).

Since September 1993, the National Institutes of Health (NIH) has funded the Women's Health Initiative (WHI) to measure the risks and benefits for heart disease, breast and colorectal cancer, and fractures among menopausal women age 50 to 79. This is the first and only large-scale, randomized, controlled clinical trial to compare the effects of hormone therapies versus placebos in healthy women. Although the WHI was intended to extend through 2005, a significant component was suddenly halted in July 2002 (after only a mean of 5.2 years of follow-up) because the risks of taking combined hormone therapy (HRT) were determined to exceed the benefits (Grady, Herrington, and Bittner et al. 2002). Although the WHI directors had informed women in 2000 and 2001 that HRT appeared to slightly increase hazards for heart attacks, strokes, and blood clots, those risks had not been considered significant enough to halt the study. In 2002, investigators found that, in addition to these slight risks, HRT also caused a slight but significant increase in the risk of invasive breast cancer which was not counterbalanced by positive but smaller reductions in the numbers of hip fractures and colorectal cancers (Grady, Harrington, and Bittner et al. 2002).[19] Letters were quickly sent to the 16,608 WHI participants who were taking combined hormone therapy, asking them to speak with their physicians regarding stopping HRT. In an article in the *Journal of the American Medical Association,* investigators conclude:

> Results from WHI indicate that the combined postmenopausal hormones . . . should not be initiated or continued for the primary prevention of CHD [coronary heart disease]. In addition, the substantial risks for cardiovascular disease and breast cancer must be weighed against the benefit for fracture in selecting from the available agents to prevent osteoporosis. (Grady, Harrington, and Bittner et al. 2002, 15)

A separate arm of the WHI study addresses health costs and benefits of ERT. This includes 10,739 women who are receiving only ERT (rather than combined therapy) because they have undergone hysterectomy. At the time the HRT arm of the WHI was terminated, the ERT component of the study was continued because the evidence did not yet indicate the same increased risks for ERT alone. Therefore, unlike the findings of the HRT arm of the study, risks were not considered to outweigh benefits. Final analysis of results of the ERT study is expected in 2005, after an average of approximately 8.5 years of follow-up. It is important to note that all of my interviews all took place prior to the announcement of the results of the HRT arm of the WHI.

While the abrupt halting of the HRT arm of the WHI study leaves women taking combined hormone therapy scared and confused, it also creates a dilemma for hysterectomized women taking only ERT. In an article in the *New York Times* (Kolata 2002), Dr. Jacques E. Rossouw, Acting Director of the WHI, declared that, with regard to ERT alone, "the risks and benefits remain unclear, but we can say there is no indication of an increased risk of breast cancer." At the time of the official announcement regarding the HRT component, Claude Lenfant, Director of the National Heart, Lung and Blood Institute of the National Institutes of Health (which is responsible for the WHI study) sent a letter to participants in the ERT arm of the WHI. This letter informed women taking ERT alone of the results of the HRT arm of the study and also stated:

> The WHI Data Safety Monitoring Board (DSMB) has recommended that your study of estrogen alone continue, because it remains uncertain whether the benefits outweigh the risks. Currently, there is no increased risk of breast cancer in women taking estrogen alone. The DSMB will continue to review the data every 6 months and we will inform you immediately if they have new recommendations. (Lenfant 2002)

This statement does not provide complete reassurance for women who continue to take ERT.

Since medical authorities had long claimed that HRT was not only safe but also beneficial for naturally menopausal women,

women taking ERT can only wonder whether extended study might establish that the safety and effectiveness of ERT for surgically menopausal women is also a fallacy. The effects of estrogen alone have not yet been proven to be safe by the WHI or other recent studies; they only remain "uncertain." This is particularly so because the combined therapy trial did not distinguish between the effects of estrogen and progestin (Grady, Herrington, and Bittner et al. 2002). Moreover, the initial WHI report did not offer conclusions regarding the positive or negative effects of hormone therapy on conditions such as gallbladder disease, diabetes, quality of life, and cognitive function, which will be examined in future reports.[20] An article addressed to physicians at the time the HRT clinical trial was halted recommends: "Although the WHI findings apply only to women with an intact uterus using combination HRT, reevaluation of the pros and cons of hormone use will be appropriate for many hysterectomized women on estrogen replacement" (Kaunitz 2002, 3). Physicians were urged to help women make decisions based on their own individual situations. For women who are on ERT, the ability to weigh risks and benefits is at least as confusing as it was at the time I interviewed respondents.

A "Balancing Act": Weighing Risks and Benefits

"What is sociologically most interesting about uncertainty is how people manage it," asserts Conrad (1987b, 7). Respondents who confronted the most difficult decisions regarding ERT were those who had familial risk factors that they were told warranted taking ERT but also familial risk factors contraindicating it. Christine and her sister faced such a dilemma because their father died of a heart attack at an early age, while their mother died of breast cancer. Although ERT had never been proven to prevent heart disease, "hundreds of thousands of women may be taking ERT/HRT because a health care practitioner told them it would prevent heart disease" (NWHN 2002, 177), and this prophylactic effect was a common perception for some time.[21] In the case of Christine and her sister, who had the same genetic histories, each made opposite decisions regarding ERT. Christine articulated the confusing situation confronted by surgically menopausal women:

> It's a great choice. And I really don't like it when the doctor sort of gave me this choice. You know? And they give it to you as if it's a choice that makes sense. I mean, it is a choice, but it's not a choice that makes sense. And it's like, would you rather drink poison or would you rather be shot?

Although the benefits for heart disease are now more unclear, the same logic applies to other possible positive or negative consequences of ERT.

Even Ann, a health educator who had exhaustively researched ERT, could find no definitive answers regarding potential future health outcomes. She justified taking exogenous estrogen by stating:

> I feel like the data on breast cancer isn't very clear vis-à-vis estrogen . . . so it feels like it's not really such a big risk. I don't feel it's any bigger risk—I don't know if I'm going to get breast cancer or not, and nobody knows. And it just seems like this doesn't make that much difference. I could get breast cancer and not take estrogen. Or I could take it and never get it . . . so I don't see any reason not to take it.

Since there is no clear rationale to take or not take ERT, Ann preferred to take it and see what would happen in the future. This was the strategy chosen by most respondents. When considering the complicated choices regarding ERT, most respondents decided to take their chances by taking the drug.

The object of medical therapy is to produce benefits that outweigh risks. Until the conclusion of the ERT arm of the WHI clinical trials, and possibly even after that, actual risks and benefits cannot be entirely clear. The precise effects of ERT on individual women are for now unknown, and they ultimately may be unknowable. This means that women will continue to receive conflicting messages, primarily because current medical information itself is so uncertain. Consistency regarding discussion of benefits and risks of ERT for surgically menopausal women not only varies among different information sources, but there are also disparities within the same sources. For example, the same short patient information pamphlet on ERT distributed by the American College of Obstetricians and Gynecologists (ACOG) contains conflicting messages. Although the authors admit to increased chances of cancer for women who take exogenous hormones for more than fifteen years, this same pamphlet also states that "[hormone] treatment may last a number of years, even decades. If you take hormones to guard against osteoporosis and heart disease [the major effects of estrogen deficiency], long term treatment is needed" (ACOG 1992a). Medical uncertainty is not unique to ERT,[22] but for many surgically menopausal women the uncertainty surrounding starting and stopping ERT is overdetermined.

In the face of medical uncertainty, decisions regarding ERT may be strongly affected by more intangible motivations than resolving or preventing physical problems. This chapter has suggested that retaining or regaining feminine gender identity was a powerful underlying motivation for a large proportion of respondents who chose to take ERT. Since other costs and benefits are so ambiguous, this rationale may assume predominant importance for many women.

4

"Badge of Femininity"?

Menstruation

Menstruation is a "badge of femininity," which may be worn in misery, pain or pride, according to the attitude of the woman.

—*J. P. Greenhill*, Office Gynecology

After that many years of bleeding, I was really thankful not to have to deal with it. And I can honestly say I don't miss that part of it at all, whatsoever. I don't miss it. I don't feel less of a woman without it.

—*Allison, a respondent*

FOR PREMENOPAUSAL women, the most obvious physical results of hysterectomy, with or without oophorectomy, are the loss of menstrual function and the ability to give birth. Although the women discussed in Chapter 3 may employ ERT to alleviate symptoms related to surgery, no respondent will ever again experience periods or childbirth. Since menstruation and childbirth are strongly associated with female gender identity, I explored the meanings of these biological functions with the women I interviewed. Menstruation is the focus of this chapter, and childbearing is the subject of the next chapter.

The Association Between Menstruation and Gender Identity

Research indicates that there is a strong association between menstruation and female gender identity (e.g., Houppert 1999; Lander

1988; Lee and Sasser-Coen 1996). For example, in her study of 165 women's menstruation experiences, Emily Martin (1992) found that respondents described menstruation as "a mark of woman-hood": "The primary positive feeling many women have about menstruation is that it *defines them as a woman*. . . . Sometimes the defining characteristic is closely linked with being able to have babies. . . . But other times the defining characteristic is equally important *apart from the potential to reproduce*" (1992, 101; emphasis added). Martin discovered that, with regard to menstruation, "over and over again, women found different ways of saying, "No I don't want to give it up, it's part of my self, part of what makes me a woman . . . it's so integral . . . it's supposed to happen" (1992, 101). As Angier asserts, "Not all women breed, but nearly all women bleed, or have bled" (1999, 95).[1] Thus, the menstruating woman is seen as a "normal" woman.

Several researchers have looked at the association between menarche (the onset of menstruation) and cultural initiation into womanhood. Sharon Golub (1983) describes the importance of physiological, psychological, and sociological issues initiated by a woman's first menstruation. Correspondingly, Martin found that most of the women she interviewed were happy at the onset of menstruation, because "part of the meaning of first menstruation is often a transition from girlhood to womanhood. . . . Mothers and sisters often greet the event with 'You're a woman now!'" (1992, 101). Angier claims, "With some exceptions, a girl loves getting her first period. She feels as though she has accomplished a great thing, willed her presence into being" (1999, 95). Other researchers (e.g., Koff, Rierdan, and Jacobsen 1981) have confirmed this observation.

Menstruation as a Connection to Other Females

A woman's menstrual period can also be viewed as symbolic of her biological tie to other women. In their study of menarche, Lee and Sasser-Coen found that "women described over and over again how, as girls, they developed camaraderie and solidarity around the [menstruation] issue" (1996, 178). One of their respondents explained, "Men don't have something to bring them to-gether, where women have this, it's shared, they understand each other" (179). Delaney, Lupton, and Toth refer to the celebration of mutual menstruation as a "heroic ritual shared by the community of women, connecting them with the rhythm of nature and each other" (1988, 168); while Martin explains more mundane ways in which menstruation brings women together. For Martin's respondents:

> A part of feeling joined together as women is feeling different from all men. . . . When women talk about the disgusting mess or the discomfort, they do so with an implicit, often unstated under-standing that there is another side to the process: it is part of what defines one as a woman, and it is something all women share, even if what we share is talking about the problem of dealing with this disgusting mess. (1992, 102–3)

Research by McClintock (1971) even found convincing evidence of "menstrual synchrony," whereby women who spend time living or working together gradually harmonize their cycles. Menstrual periods evidently can constitute a symbolic and material bond be-tween women.

The Connection Between Female Gender Identity and Menstrual Problems

Dysmenorrhea is the medical term for painful menstrual periods. According to Lander (1988), researchers who have attempted to discover correlations between femininity and dysmenorrhea have found conflicting results. Some studies demonstrate that women who identify strongly with traditional feminine characteristics ex-perience more painful menstrual periods; others have shown the opposite; and a third set of studies reveal no association between personality type and dysmenorrhea.

Woods (1986) investigated whether traditional feminine social-ization was related to the extent of menstrual problems that women suffered. The only correlation she discovered was that the women who had the most annoying periods held the strongest negative attitudes toward menstruation. "Thus," she determines, "it appears that menstrual attitudes are not merely a product of socialization but also a function of women's experiences with symptoms that disrupt their lives" (126). Lander refers to this as "the reality effect" (1988, 177). These analyses imply that menstruation carries ambivalent meanings for women and points the way to an understanding of why the ending of menstruation may also be an ambivalent experience.

Cessation of Menstruation and Gender Identity

If menarche signifies an individual's initiation into womanhood, does the cessation of menstruation mean that she is no longer a woman? The significance of menstruation as a symbol of female normality makes this a plausible question. Some researchers (e.g., Kaufert 1982; Rogers 1997) claim that natural menopause can present gender identity problems for older women. However, although naturally menopausal women may have some doubts regarding their womanhood, they can be reassured by recognizing that they are going through a natural female transition. I expected that women whose menstrual careers were cut short by surgery would have more serious regrets. This expectation, which later proved erroneous, had been fostered by some prominent previous research on hysterectomy.

Drelich and Bieber (1958) conducted probably the most often-cited research regarding menstruation and hysterectomy. They studied the experiences of twenty-three patients who had undergone hysterectomy for benign and malignant reasons, and investigated the women's attitudes and emotional reactions before and after surgical removal of their uteruses. Drelich and Bieber concluded:

> Menstruation is a uniquely feminine experience and its imminent termination, as an obvious consequence of hysterectomy, was given considerable attention by the women studied. . . . [D]espite the frequent negative attitudes expressed by many women towards the symptoms which accompany their menstrual periods, *the majority of women feel primarily positive feelings toward the menstrual function as a whole and deplore the loss of this valued activity.* (1958, 324; emphasis added)

Almost thirty years later, Rosenhand (1984) revisited this contention and confirmed that women generally viewed menstruation as a source of well-being and a positively valued function.

At the time of their study, Drelich and Bieber (1958) objected to medical literature emphasizing the negative attitudes toward menstruation while ignoring the positive value placed on menstruation by many women. This has certainly not been the case in the last twenty to thirty years as seen in the more recent research that discusses a wide variety of positive aspects regarding menstruation.[2]

Respondents' Perceptions of Menarche as a Measure of Female Normality

"What women remember about their experiences surrounding and including menarche and their subsequent bodily histories provides insight into what was most salient about the event not only when it occurred, but as it is reconsidered over time," Lee and Sasser-Coen emphasize (1996, 38). Thus, menarche is symbolically significant. My aim in asking respondents about their menarche experiences was to learn more about how they interpreted the connection between gender identity and menstruation from their earliest experiences.

When I asked each respondent at what point she initially realized that she was female, almost all reported that recognition had occurred with their first periods. Regardless of whether menstruation caused them joy, pride, pain, or embarrassment, menarche signified the moment of becoming "a woman." Most were informed of their new status by significant others. For example, when Lupe told her Puerto Rican grandmother that she had gotten her menstrual period, the older woman informed everyone, "The rooster has sung!" Lupe explained that this meant that she had become a woman.

Menarche was a momentous occasion in the life cycle of many respondents. When she finally got her period, Deborah explained, "I was relieved! It was a victory! . . . Because I knew that this had to do with maturing. And it was what was expected normally. I don't remember how much I understood about the fact that at that point you would be able to have a child." Accordingly, even before they had a clear understanding that menstruation was related to fertility, many respondents saw menarche as a sign of normality, of being like other women. Respondents discussed aspects of menarche as a measuring stick for gender identity according to several themes, including age at menarche, connection with other females, and recognition as females by their fathers.

Age at Menarche

In general, respondents reported either that they had gotten their first periods "early" (between ages 9 and 11½) or "late" (between ages 12 and 17). It was unusual for women to say that they had gotten their first periods "on time." A girl's age at menarche was seen, not as an objective measure, but in comparison to sisters or friends. Those respondents who started their menstrual periods earlier than their peers were generally embarrassed, afraid of being teased, and often hid their "secret" until others joined them. Sunny, for example, was "mortified" when she began to menstruate at age 9: "Very early—way too early." She kept it a secret and described herself as "a tomboy with pads—bleeding in elementary school—it was a lot for a 9-year-old to feel." Those respondents who started their periods later than other girls they knew were also embarrassed and tried to hide the fact that they had not yet menstruated. Ann told me:

> Well, I got it pretty late. I didn't get my period until I was 14½, which I think everybody else I knew, at least to the extent that they were telling the truth, had already gotten theirs. . . . I thought there was something wrong with me.

Thus, menarche symbolized a normative female status for respondents.

Connection with Other Females

Several women reminisced about how they felt closer to mothers, girlfriends, or sisters at the time of their first menstruation. Terry, who got her first menstrual period at 12½, told me that she was "dying for it." Not only did she have four older sisters, but her best friend had started to menstruate six months earlier: "I just couldn't wait 'cause I wanted to be part of that." Terry stated that when she told her mother she had started her period, "She sort of hugged me and said, 'Oh that's wonderful. Now you're a *woman!*' And I said, 'I hate it. I wanted it, but now I hate it. It's a mess!'" However, Terry found that even the "mess" created a bond with other females. As she continued to explain, "In talking to my girl-friends, then I realized that they all felt the same way too. And as I continued to have my period, I was more included with my older sisters, and they would sort of moan and groan together." This mutual complaining appears to be part of the bonding that often takes place between women regarding the common experience of menstruation (Martin 1992).

Recognition as Females by Fathers

Although mothers and other female relatives figured prominently in respondents' accounts, a number of respondents spontaneously volunteered that their fathers had been very close and helpful to them at the time of menarche. For example, when Madison ran into her parents' room to tell them she had gotten her first period, her mother only told her to clean her sheets, whereas her father said proudly, "Oh, our little girl is growing up."

Several women repeated stories describing how their fathers, rather than their female relatives, were the first to buy them sanitary supplies. Christine's father found her crying on the day of her first period because she was humiliated that her Italian-born aunt had insisted that she wear rags to soak up the menstrual flow ("If it's good enough for me, it's good enough for you"). Christine told me that, despite their poverty, "somehow my father just went to the store and bought it [sanitary napkins]."

Some fathers even went further than buying sanitary supplies. Gloria's mother never explained menstruation to her before she got her first period, and she was grateful that her father came into the bathroom with a sanitary napkin and a belt and told her "what to do with it." Allison's mother wouldn't let her wear tampons as a young teen because she thought that would make her promiscuous. When Allison complained to her father about the mess her period made, he not only convinced her mother to let her wear tampons, but he also stood outside the bathroom door reading the manual while she practiced inserting her first one.

None of the women who talked about their fathers' involvement in their menarche interpreted this as inappropriately intrusive. Respondents' experiences demonstrate that the onset of menstruation is not only a time for girls to bond with other females. Other research on menarche (Lee and Sasser-Coen 1996) found that separation and secrecy occurs between the newly menstruating girl and males. Several respondents did discuss their need to hide their periods from boys and men in their lives. However, as the stories told above illustrate, at the time of menarche, girls' relationships as females can also be solidified with their fathers, usually the most significant males in young girls' lives.

Negative Aspects of Menstruation as Initiation into Womanhood

EMBARRASSMENT, AWKWARDNESS, AND RULES FOR FEMALE BEHAVIOR. In addition to the positive aspects of womanhood to which respondents were introduced at menarche, they also recalled initiation into negative aspects of female gender identity. For example, in recognition of family tradition, Page's mother slapped her face when she got her period at 9 years old and told her, "First blood is bad blood, you have to slap it away." Other respondents, like 12-year-old Janet, who bled through white shorts while at a coed social gathering, described being embarrassed by their first periods. Women also discussed how self-conscious they felt about "all the equipment" they were compelled to employ during their periods. This was particularly true for Charlotte, who had to use torn sheets and rags instead of Kotex for the first years she menstruated. Even those women who wore sanitary napkins complained that they were uncomfortable. As Gloria griped, "What a contraption—like a mattress between your legs—awful." Allison claimed the pads "crinkled when you walked," and Barbara explained that she could only wear certain clothing while menstruating because the belt and pad were "chunky in front" and "would stick out." These experiences sent respondents strong messages regarding the embarrassment and awkwardness that can be associated with female identity.

Many women also talked about new social restrictions that were placed on them when they reached menarche. Several were cautioned that they could not go swimming while they were menstruating, and Ernestine was told by the orphanage matron that she'd "go crazy" if she washed her hair during her period. Isabella discussed certain taboos she was supposed to follow during menstruation, including "don't drink lemons, pineapple, coconuts; don't climb trees; don't touch flowers; don't touch small babies; don't go in the water because it will make the waves come higher." As Gloria put it, there were "*too many* don'ts."

Respondents didn't necessarily believe these prohibitions were valid and generally resisted them. For example, Ernestine felt good that she had rebelled by washing her hair during her menstrual periods despite the matron's warnings and laughed, "Maybe I *did* go crazy, but I don't *care!*" In addition to restrictions during menstruation, several women faced new restraints on their general behavior simply because they had made the transition to become menstruating women. Christine told me that at the onset of menstruation she was told she "couldn't do this, this, this. . . . Now you can't jump rope anymore, can't skate, can't ride a bicycle." Even if respondents opposed them, these restrictions reinforced their awareness that their status as "women who menstruate" required them to conform to female norms. This further strengthened the connection between menstruation and gender role.

ENTRY INTO ADULT FEMALE SEXUALIZATION. "Menarche marks a simultaneous entry into adult womanhood and adult female sexualization," suggests Lee (1998, 84). Many respondents found that menarche transformed them into "dangerous" sexual beings. For example, Stella told me that her mother explained, "'You're going to bleed someday, and that means you're a woman.' But don't let no man stick his pee-pee inside of your pee-pee.' And that was the end of it. And I was like, '*What* is she talking about?'" Menarche, as a symbol of fertility, was often a time that respondents were instilled with a fear of premarital pregnancy. For example, Andrea was proud when she got her first menstrual period and told her mother, "Oh, Mom, just think, I can have a baby now!" Her mother slapped Andrea's face, yelled, "Don't you ever say that again!" and walked away from her. When Penny reached menarche, her mother told her, "'Now stay away from boys—whenever you are near boys, keep your legs crossed.'" Penny assumed that, as someone who menstruated, she could now become pregnant through a boy's kiss. Similarly, when Charlotte's aunt told her that getting her period meant she was now a woman and that "you're not to let no boy touch you," she thought that she could now get pregnant just by being touched, which was a frightening concept.

In sum, respondents' perceptions of the connection between menstruation and female gender identity carried both positive and negative connotations. The contradictions regarding menstruation, which began in menarche, anticipated the ambivalence respondents would also experience at the end of their menstrual careers.

Missed Aspects of Menstruation

As discussed above, previous research regarding hysterectomy implies that women who have undergone hysterectomy regret the premature termination of menstruation. According to some researchers (Kaufert 1982; Rogers 1997), even the cessation of menstruation at natural menopause can be felt as a loss of femininity. Did any respondents express the sentiment that they missed menstruation? The three major aspects that these women regretted losing were: the use of menstrual cyclicity as a regulator of their daily lives; a feeling of connection to other menstruating women; and the redeployment of menstruation for their own emotional needs.

Menstrual Cyclicity as a Regulator

A few women, although generally relieved to be free of menstrual periods, did say that they felt they had lost a sense of cyclicity in their lives. This confirms findings by other researchers (Drelich and Bieber 1958; Rosenhand 1984; Sloan 1978). Most respondents, regardless of length of cycle, recalled how "regular" their periods had been. They used terms like "clockwork," "consistent," "right on time," "precise," and "predictable" as well as "very regular," "pretty regular," "real regular," and "regular to the second" to describe how they had been able to plan when they would begin to menstruate each month. Those few women whose cycles had been "irregular" thought that this component of their menstrual periods was problematic. This again indicates how menstruation can be seen as a measure of normality for women. Care of the self during menstruation is a cultural practice that reinforces femininity.

Although it can be liberating to be free of menstrual periods, some women can also be disoriented by the loss of this "normal" regulation of time and space. In an essay describing her own experience of hysterectomy, novelist Lynne Sharon Schwartz laments:

> You can't truthfully say you miss menstruation, but how will you learn to keep track of time, the seasons of the month? A wall calendar? But how will you know inside? Can it be that time will feel all the same, not coming to fruition and dropping the fruit, no filling and subsiding, moist and dry, moving towards and moving away from? (1987, 51)

Several respondents confirmed that they missed this aspect of menstruation. For example, Alice described her feelings as follows:

> Well, all these years . . . I had regulated myself. If I started a diet, or if I . . . my whole life had been regulated by my period and grounded by that too . . . it was a place to start, and it was a place to end the month. No matter what else was in the month, *that* was in the month. So it started and ended and then began again, so

you had that cycle that somehow grounded you. . . . I don't know. It was psychological. You knew you had your period, you knew that for that many days you bled, and it was like I would start things. I could rely on that being my monthly cycle. . . . It was a renewal. . . . But when I didn't have it any more, I felt up in the air. Like, "What do I do now?" For so many years I had sort of inadvertently made my schedule around this, however it worked, whatever I did. And then I didn't have it any more. I was thrilled that I didn't have the smell and the overburdened . . . that was lovely to get rid of that mess. But you don't remember that after— what you remember is that there's nothing. What you're faced with there's nothing—I was faced with nothing to regulate whatever psychological thing I had always done for so many years. So I was angry that I hadn't understood that better.

Although Alice was the most vociferous regarding this loss of life rhythm, other respondents mentioned it as well. As Terry described it:

I think our cycles bind us all together, and I think there is also a connection with nature with it. I mean, you can't help but—I couldn't help but, on a monthly basis, feel a rhythm of life going on in my body. And whether you call it—the tides, or the moons, or the changes—there was some sort of connection, you know?[3]

Some women who retained their ovaries after hysterectomy still claimed to feel this sense of cyclicity even though they no longer menstruated. Bernadette told me, "I feel like I'm going to get my period, but I don't." When questioned further, she told me, "Just like my stomach, like what I had before, I know—like right now, I should be having it . . . because this is the time of the month I always have it, and I feel like I should be having it right now."

Connection to Other Females

A few women believed that they had lost another kind of connection, not only to their own bodily cycles but also to other women. For example, Janet lamented, "I wasn't a member of the club anymore." She particularly regretted that when her daughter reached menarche she could not share the experience of having menstrual periods with her: "We can't confide and commiserate with each other in that sort of women-to-woman bond." In contrast, Brooke was one of several respondents mentioned in Chapter 2 who retained their ovaries after hysterectomy and believed that this preserved their hormonal cycles despite their lack of menstrual bleeding. "In some ways . . . I still identify with other women . . . when people sit and talk about going through PMS, I can still identify, I can still talk about it, I can still be part of the conversation," she explained.

Redeployment of Menstruation for Emotional Needs

Several researchers (e.g., Lee 1994; Martin 1992; Lee and Sasser-Coen 1996) describe the ways in which women often redeploy menstrual periods for their own interests. A few respondents mentioned missing some otherwise negative aspects of menstruation for this reason. Some women referred to times in their youth when they had pretended to have their periods in order to "get away with" things. Others discussed how their periods had sometimes offered them a welcome time-out from their stressful adult lives. Yvonne, for instance, disclosed that when she had bad menstrual cramps, she would lie down and rest, which provided her with a needed break that she no longer feels justified to take. Donna told me that she would get "very crampy, very bloated, very irritable" on the day she got her period, and, she claimed, "I used to save any task that I dreaded doing because I had to confront somebody or be assertive. I would save it for that day!" She elaborated:

> So I would spend the day bitching everybody out that I needed to bitch out [laughing]. . . . It took me a while to figure that out, but I started figuring out that I could put up with a lot less bullshit and get a lot further on that day of the month with some situations. . . . If I had a repairman who had screwed up or something like that, and I knew I was going to start my period in two or three days, I would wait. . . . And he wouldn't know what hit him, you know? . . . And I think . . . I was just not sweet, you know? . . . I

think it was just that I wasn't in the mood to be polite. And some-times, at other times of the month, I might be so polite that I wasn't able to express what I wanted done, but I just seemed to be able to do it more to the point.

Martin (1992) explains that this premenstrual expression of rage is a release from cultural expectations that women should gener-ally control their anger; Shuttle and Redgrove assert that this is "a moment of truth which will not sustain lies" (1978, 58). Donna is one respondent whose only regret about ceasing to menstruate is that she no longer feels those monthly "moments of truth."

Relief as Primary Reaction

Although some women in this study did miss certain aspects of menstruation, the primary reaction of respondents was almost unanimous relief that they no longer menstruated. They repeat-edly voiced sentiments like "I don't miss my period at all" and "Thank God that's over!" Based on previous research regarding hysterectomy, this reaction by respondents was unexpected. How-ever, it is important to view this finding in the context of the tremendous pain and bleeding that most respondents had experi-enced, some since menarche, others in the months and years right before their surgery.

Pain

For most of the women I interviewed, their menstrual and pre-menstrual pain had been overwhelming as well as highly resistant to treatment:

I had horrible nightmares because I cramped up so bad every month. . . . I suffered so badly, the pain was so bad no matter what I did—not hot water bottles, not Midol—I tried everything I pos-sibly could—I just lay on my stomach or rolled up on the floor with my feet in the air, rubbing my stomach—Darvon finally worked good—until I started vomiting them up—I was always miserable—a very miserable person. (Penny)

I had to sit out phys. ed. in high school. I had really, really, heavy, heavy periods—cramps so bad I could hardly move. I couldn't walk—they got progressively worse—long, long periods—I stayed home from work for 23 days [in one year]—with terrible pain in my lower abdomen and back. . . . I couldn't stand the pain . . . felt faint. I would rather have taken a beating than to have my period, or done anything short of getting pregnant all the time, to not have a period. (Letitia)

I had a lot of pain from the beginning—couldn't walk—I was screaming, crying, couldn't sleep—crazy—took Excedrin. . . . [I] couldn't sleep but stayed in bed. After my first baby the pain went away for two years, but then it got even worse. (Isabella)

I had migraine headaches—had to come home from work or school—couldn't do anything. I was nauseous and vomiting—I could not function. (Margie)

I had bad periods from the beginning. The cramps were debilitating. . . . I took Motrin . . . nothing worked. . . . Aspirin and coffee and heating pads. . . . They got progressively worse—I was unable to function with my period! (Susan)

Heavy Bleeding

Menorrhagia is the medical term for excessive gynecological bleeding. Several women were debilitated not only by pain but by heavy bleeding as well, which was commonly the ultimate rationale for their hysterectomies. Many women are bothered by the complications created by menstrual blood, and three-quarters of the women that Lee (1998) interviewed reported embarrassment over staining due to menstrual bleeding. However, stories about bleeding from the women I interviewed went far beyond mere embarrassment. The following examples demonstrate the extent of their distress:

I would bleed up to ten days. . . . One time a friend saw me and got really scared and called my husband to tell him I was hemorrhaging—she couldn't believe it was normal for me. (Joyce)

Once I was in line at the supermarket and I saw it on the floor—
devastating. It would come with such force—such a gush—all over
my clothes—horrible, horrible. Every time I had a period it was
like I was afraid to go someplace. I'd only wear black. I tended not
to wear pants because it was easier to lift than pull. . . . I hated
changing the sheets—I'd put a towel down instead. . . . It made
me feel unclean—always blood. . . . I was afraid to stand near people. (Joy)

The majority of respondents talked about the great extent to
which their activities were circumscribed by pain or excessive
bleeding. In view of these circumstances, the end of menstruation came as a great relief, as expressed by Barbara:

I could only go a certain distance the summer before the hysterectomy. I had a pad on most of the summer. . . . This [being
without periods] is wonderful . . . this is *wonderful!!*

Belief That Quality of Life Is Better Without Menstrual Periods
The vast majority of respondents firmly stated that they did not
miss their menstrual periods. Stella explained that her first
thought upon waking after hysterectomy was "Well, no more
pain every month. Fine!" Most other respondents echoed this
thought:

Frankly, it's such a relief not to have monthly periods and pain—
for me it was a *godsend.* I have been so much happier since then—
don't miss it at all. (Susan)

[My period] was a pain in the ass. . . . I always felt that it was a disturbance and a hassle in my life. I never thought 'What a wonderful thing, to be a woman!' No. Never. . . . To me, this was a life-
long dream, to not have my period any more. (Brooke)

I was thrilled in every way conceivable not to have periods. . . . I
felt happier because I wasn't bleeding anymore. (Sunny)

Not having periods is the best in the world—I never went any
place where I ever felt comfortable when I had a period. (Joy)

To be honest with you, I love not having my period—I feel freer—
There was a nice piece to that—I just enjoy the *freedom*. (Sarah)

Oh, my god! I was so happy. I was so happy. All that grief! I just
feel so wonderful. I don't miss it one bit, not a bit! . . . I thought I
would do a ritual once month where I would observe it in its absence . . . and thought about retaining my connection with the
moon, and blah, blah, blah. . . . I never even think about it, not
once. . . . I feel like I've got my life back! And I didn't feel like I was
giving anything in exchange. It was just that I got something I
should have had all along, which was a quality of life that allowed
me to do what I needed to do. And my period was taking that
away from me. (Andrea)

For these women, menstruation was much more serious than the
"friendly monthly nuisance" described by Delaney, Lupton, and
Toth (1988, 4). Their menstrual periods were viewed as invasions
that threatened the quality of their lives.

Beliefs Regarding the Normality of Female Suffering

Most respondents told me that they ignored severe pain and copious bleeding for long periods of time because they were taught
that it was "normal" for women to bleed and be in pain. For instance, although "completely debilitated by her periods," Yvonne
"just figured it was part of life, of being a girl." Page didn't realize
how incapacitating her periods really were until her doctor had
her keep a diary and she realized that "I had a month where I had
only two or three good days." Most respondents who did complain to doctors, family members, friends, or co-workers were
often patronized with unhelpful advice like "Have a positive attitude . . . if you think you'll have problems, you will" (Kelly);
"Everybody goes through it—throw-up and you'll feel better"
(Margie); "You must be making it up!" (Ann); or "If you think this
hurts—just wait until you have a baby!" (Christine). This kind of
commentary, as well as the assumption that "other women have
it so much worse," which I heard from several respondents,
caused women to deny pain and hemorrhaging for long periods
of time. They were usually repeatedly told there was nothing

wrong with them physically and were made to feel that they were emotionally unbalanced.

When Leigh finally summoned the courage to tell her doctor about her horrible pain and copious bleeding, he responded that she probably had "a very low pain threshold." During surgery, however, it became obvious that she had extensive endometriosis, which she had been able to endure only because her pain threshold was actually very high. Similarly, Terry complained of tortuous periods for years and was told to "grin and bear it." When her gynecologist finally did a laparoscopy after a ruptured ovarian cyst, he was "absolutely shocked," she told me. "And I can clearly remember him almost apologizing. . . . He said, 'I never realized that your menstrual cramps were as bad as what they were!' I said, 'You know what? I never really did either!'"

The expectation that all women should consider pain and hemorrhaging just a matter of course was strongly instilled in respondents. Even *after* they underwent hysterectomies and oophorectomies in order to stop their own great pain and profuse bleeding, several of them continued to believe that women should suffer in silence. A case in point was Frances, who informed me that she convinced her doctor she needed surgery "because I was sick of bleeding." She also told me that, as a child, she had persuaded her mother's doctor to end the older woman's pain through hysterectomy. However, Frances still believed that women in general should just "grin and bear" their periods because "pain is only mind over matter." Although thrilled that she had a hysterectomy and oophorectomy at 49 so that she wouldn't have to wait for her fibroids to shrink at natural menopause, Frances emphatically explained, "You do have a period, and yes, the best way to deal with it is as a natural way of life. . . . Women only suffer with their periods if they *want* to suffer with their periods!"

In great detail, Page described the terrible monthly pain she experienced prior to hysterectomy. Yet, in a memo she sent to me the day after our interview, she expressed concern that "women use 'monthly excuses' to avoid unpleasant situations . . . and to avoid responsibility by 'copping out.'" Page admitted that she herself had "fallen victim to this" and wrote: "At times when stress is overwhelming (from entirely different sources), it is easy to blow something off when an outsider offers a reasonable escape. 'Don't worry about it (dear, honey). I know it's that time of the month.'" Thus, most respondents accepted the belief that it is "normal" for menstruating women to suffer. It is striking that these women were strongly socialized to deny excessive pain and bleeding to the extent that they suffered for long periods of time until finally forced to undergo major surgery for relief. More startling is the fact that even after this surgery some respondents continued to support oppressive arguments regarding the normality of female misery that was directed against other women who suffer as they once did.

Disassociation with Menstruating Women

The menstrual pain and heavy bleeding that almost all respondents endured were so severe that these negative experiences far overshadowed any positive association they might have had regarding women's common experience of menstruation. Contrary to expressing remorse that they no longer identified with other women because they had ceased menstruating, most respondents acknowledged that they pity women who still have menstrual periods. Moreover, their narratives demonstrate that they deliberately sought to disassociate themselves from the suffering that they perceived is a normal condition for all menstruating women:

> I have two boys, and I'm usually with a man, so I'm not used to seeing pads and Tampax and stuff like that. But now, in the women's shelter, it's like "Oh yeah, I remember those days!" I'm glad that part of it is over. (Wendy)

> Well, it's weird. . . . When [her life partner] is acting premenstrual and having all this stuff . . . I find myself saying, "Oh, you must be premenstrual, you're acting really weird." . . . Well, I'm glad it's not me. I hated it. I'm happy not to be premenstrual or have cramps or any of that stuff any more. (Ann)

I feel really sorry for them [women who still menstruate]. I do. I feel like I'm in this blissful place and it will be years before they know about it. (Andrea)

Thus, for the overwhelming majority of respondents, the premature termination of their menstrual cycles through hysterectomy did not constitute a regretted loss to their subjective female gender identities.

Women's reactions to menarche, menstruation, and the end of menstruation were bound up in both their own physical experiences of these phenomena and the cultural and social implications that these female occurrences bear. While their own previous pain and bleeding led them to feel physical relief, the symbolic meaning that associated this suffering with female normality promoted positive feelings regarding their ability to transcend the menstrual aspect of gender identity.

Respondents' predominant lack of remorse over premature menstrual cessation contrasts strongly with regretted losses that many of these same women relate to other biological functions, including childbearing and sexuality. These conclusions affirm that it is crucial to recognize that hysterectomy does not have universal effects on the complex phenomenon of female gender identity.

5

"Women's Work"?

Motherhood and Gender Identity

Motherhood is, after all, woman's great and incomparable work.

—*Edward Carpenter, "Woman in Freedom"*

The feminist movement would reject all theories which would tie the definition of a woman to her sexuality and her reproductive role. But . . . the concentration of the women's health movement on issues of reproduction and childbirth has tended to reinforce this model rather than overturn it.

—*Patricia A. Kaufert, "Myth and the Menopause"*

SINCE HYSTERECTOMY ends a woman's ability to bear children, this surgery highlights the highly complex relationship between reproduction and gender identity. Traditionally, a "normal" woman has been expected to fulfill the mothering role, and any deviation from this is therefore regarded as suspect: "Motherhood is often perceived as the quintessence of womanhood. The everyday tasks of mothering are taken to be "natural" expressions of femininity, and the routine care of home and children are seen to provide opportunities for women to express and reaffirm their gendered relation to men and the world" (Coltrane 1989, 473).

The debate regarding whether desire for motherhood is innate or learned has never been settled; the best evidence suggests that both biology and socialization are important components of maternal feelings (Hrdy 1999). While the ability to give birth is a physical capability for most women, the understanding that *all* women must mother is a cultural expectation.

Feminist theories regarding the connection between motherhood and womanhood are highly contentious. While some theorists argue vehemently that women have been exploited by their identification as mothers, others view motherhood as an important and valued characteristic of womanhood (Chodorow and Contratto 1982; Lorber et al. 1981). Reproductive capability has been problematic when used as a justification to force women into nurturing roles while limiting alternative possibilities. However, many women see the unique ability to give birth as a source of female strength.

The Nature of Nurture

Most of the women I interviewed accepted strong cultural beliefs that motherhood is an essential component of women's identity. Loss of reproductive organs thus created insecurity regarding gender identity for these women. For example, Letitia, mother of three, told me that her first thoughts after hysterectomy were that she was "not a real woman. . . . I think it's . . . all of a sudden you're not reproducing, and you were put here for reproducing and all that stuff. Even though I didn't plan to have any more kids." Other respondents' reactions were somewhat more nuanced, but the majority perceived that they had lost an important "natural" connection between being a woman and being a mother.

Since Brooke did not believe that maternal desire was a "natural" phenomenon, she was surprised at the emotional loss she experienced following surgery. Before undergoing hysterectomy at age 34, Brooke's gynecologist suggested that she think about whether she ever wanted to give birth. Consequently, she did some reading in self-help books about the possible emotional effects of losing reproductive organs. Nonetheless, since the books referred only to heterosexual women who had husbands, Brooke assumed that these warnings did not apply to her as a lesbian who had never previously desired pregnancy. Prior to hysterectomy, Brooke believed that her uterus was as "insignificant" as her gall bladder, which had already been removed with no emotional consequences. Therefore, she was shocked when she became extremely depressed approximately six months after her hysterectomy:

> I realized I was a woman, and I realized I wasn't going to be able to have kids anymore, and even though I didn't want [children], all of a sudden I felt myself going through what all the books said the heterosexual women went through. I was going through it. I felt that I was missing part of my womanhood because I couldn't have kids.

Brooke attempted to analyze her post-surgery feelings, and came to the following conclusions:

> I think that was all about society. Even though I verbally said I wasn't a part of what society said I was, I think all my life, as growing up a girl, I was told I was going to have babies and do this. And I think psychologically I was mourning not having a uterus without even knowing it. . . . I was shocked. I was very shocked and angry. I was angry at society because I was forced into this mourning. I was forced into this. It was like "God damn it. . . ." It was bullshit. . . . I felt like there was a psychological, societal force that was at play that I did not choose. Because I was raised in the way I was . . . .

Despite her understanding of the social origins of her suffering, Brooke told me that she still went through a deep sense of deprivation. Like Brooke, for many respondents the inability to fulfill maternal expectations was considered a loss of womanhood, regardless of whether they believed that maternal desire was socialized or inborn.

Infertility and Female Identity

Several researchers (e.g., Greil 1991a and b; Miall 1986; 1994) have found that infertility can produce feelings of failure that precipitate what Matthews and Matthews refer to as "'identity shock'" (1986, 645). Greil (1997) concludes that infertility is a much more stressful experience for women than for men due to social constructions that equate female identity with giving birth. Obviously, women for whom motherhood is particularly salient will be most affected.

A number of studies (e.g., Dreilich and Beiber 1958; Kaltreider et al. 1979; Roeske 1979) have stressed that hysterectomy may be particularly distressing for women who are childless or premenopausal because they may not have fulfilled their childbearing potential. However, Deanette Palmer suggests that loss of childbearing potential may no longer be a serious consequence of hysterectomy since motherhood has become a less significant component of identity for contemporary women: "Historically, a woman's self-esteem has been derived primarily from her reproductive functions. . . . Currently, social changes have increased women's expectations of fulfillment outside of motherhood. In fact, the potential for an increased number of sources for status and self-esteem may change the emotional meaning of hysterectomy" (1984, 5; see also Roeske 1979).

My data do not support this conclusion. The preponderance of women I interviewed, regardless of whether they had other sources of fulfillment, still placed considerable importance on childbearing. On the contrary, I found evidence to support Howard and Hollander's claim that "despite the multiplicity of roles that women may now inhabit, many professional women may still see bearing and caring for children as 'a way of constructing femininity'" (1997, 154). In fact, loss of the ability to bear children through hysterectomy may even be a greater problem for contemporary women than it was for previous generations. Since more women currently delay childbearing in order to fulfill other roles, they are therefore more likely to be childless at the time of hysterectomy. Despite Palmer's claim, this may result in more rather than less severe emotional reactions for contemporary women who lose their ability to bear children through hysterectomy. Most respondents expressed feelings that female identity is at least partially contingent on achieving motherhood. Thus, undergoing hysterectomy threatened that identity.

Women's Reactions to Loss of Fertility

No Regrets: Some Childless Women

The importance that the vast majority of respondents placed on the ability to reproduce meant that their hysterectomies created emotional gender crises, especially for those who had never given birth. There were only a few exceptions to this, and these were all women who had previously resolved that they did not wish to produce biological children and maintained that resolve following surgery. For example, Frances told me that, although she had spent her life working with children, she never had an interest in having her own. Despite her own mother's comment that it was "unnatural" not to become a mother, Frances felt that being a parent is "the biggest job in the world," and she was not prepared to make the necessary "sacrifices." Amber explained that she was "just so preoccupied" with her career that she didn't think about having a family, while Andrea's experience of caring for a dying younger sister prompted her to feel "sort of relieved when she found out she would be infertile" because she "wouldn't have to risk losing a child."

The most extreme example of a childless woman who had no regrets was Leigh, who, conversely, viewed infertility as "an amazing side benefit" to surgery. She had always expected to have children someday until, when she was in her early twenties, she recognized that she wanted to "own" her life and that parenthood would "be a block" to that. Having seen the struggles of her single mother and the "never-ending work" of her aunt, who had a mentally retarded child, Leigh decided that she didn't have enough patience to be a "natural mom." By the time she married in her early thirties, Leigh felt that she had "maybe room in my life for a partner, but not for children." She was relieved that not only did her husband have a daughter from a previous marriage but also that he was probably now sterile as the result of an illness. Prior to hysterectomy and bs-o, Leigh had felt that her husband's family placed her under "enormous pressure" to produce a child. She was angry that they couldn't accept her choice not to have children and perceived that they always expected her to change her mind.

According to Leigh, the "social implications" of her surgery were "enormously positive." The family "went into the pity mode" because she was newly married and only 34 years old and would now never be able to give birth. Leigh was relieved that she was now "off the hook" about her choice not to parent; family members viewed her hysterectomy as "a deep-seated tragedy" and interpreted Leigh's protestations about not wanting children as "bravery." This confirms findings by Matthews and Matthews (1986, 646–47), who indicate that people who are involuntarily infertile "may find themselves receiving far greater acceptance than the voluntarily childless, whose justifications are frequently seen by others as self-serving and are unlikely to rouse the elements of pity that the involuntarily childless frequently receive." Leigh was content that the family pressure to produce a child "simply stopped" because relatives felt that as a result of her hysterectomy it was now a "sensitive subject." Nine years after surgery, Leigh told me that she still had no regrets about never giving birth. Her relationship with her stepdaughter, whom she has known since she was age 3, has always been as an "adult friend," never as a parent, and that is sufficient for her.

Previously Acknowledged Regrets: Some Childless Women

In discussing natural menopause, Notman (1993, 244) points out that for many childless women "coming to terms with childlessness may not coincide with the actual cessation of menses" but may be in the context of other life circumstances. Similarly, for some respondents events that preceded their hysterectomies had confirmed that they would never give birth. Charlotte, for example, told me that she had more miscarriages than she could count and was unable to produce a child despite several gynecological surgeries. By the time she had one ovary removed many years prior to her hysterectomy, she had already realized that the likelihood of her getting pregnant and giving birth was very small. She explained that she and her husband continued trying to get her pregnant, but, she said, "We just didn't try as hard."

Susan felt that "probably the most painful aspect of my life is that I was not able to have children." However, at the time she had married her present husband, they had reached an agreement that they would not have children because he was eleven years older, already had two children in high school, and didn't want to "start over with little ones." Susan explained:

> I really frankly think that the emotional aspect had come and gone before I had the operation [hysterectomy]. . . . I couldn't have children. But since I had already come to that decision, because in order to marry Mark, that was the decision I had to make. . . . I guess I just chose that over what might have been.

Thus, Susan did not interpret her hysterectomy at age 41 as the only cause of her childlessness.

No Regrets: Some Women with Biological Children

A few respondents with biological children had previously determined that they did not want any more. Some of these women had their fallopian tubes tied as a form of birth control.[1] However, the preponderance of women who already had biological children were, like their childless peers, disappointed to lose their fertility through hysterectomy. Joy and Catherine were the most conspicuous of the very few exceptions I found; they were relieved that surgery had rendered them infertile.

Joy nearly had an abortion because her third child was an "accident." Several years later, when she suffered from extremely heavy periods due to fibroid tumors, her gynecologist asked if she ever intended to have more children. Joy told him, "No, I think I would be very happy *not* to have to worry about becoming pregnant." She has never regretted her decision to have a hysterectomy and believes that her family's quality of life and her own career benefited because she did not have additional children.

Catherine, who had been a strict Catholic, had five children by the time she was 31. She explained that she had been very sick during her last two pregnancies and her labor had been prolonged for several days. After her youngest child was born, Catherine was "so frantic and so paranoid that I was absolutely petrified that I would get pregnant again 'cause I had been so sick." Catherine explained that her obstetrician had ten children of his own, was a devout Catholic, and "his hands had been knighted by the Pope," so that he never mentioned the possibility of tubal ligation or even birth control to her. On the other hand, her family doctor was alarmed about the state of her health and informed Catherine, "You *cannot* have another child. You'll *die!*" While she finally agreed to use a diaphragm, Catherine was still afraid she would become pregnant, and she began to have anxiety attacks. Very shortly after her fifth child was born, she started getting very heavy periods, her family doctor found endometriosis, and she had a hysterectomy. Catherine was thrilled to become infertile and believes that it probably saved her life.

The Despair of Childless Women

Nearly all of the childless women I interviewed were distraught rather than relieved that they were now infertile. Leigh, who, as discussed above had been mollified by her infertility, compared herself to an acquaintance who had a hysterectomy despite desperately wanting to have children. She felt that the "devastating" problems this other woman suffered following hysterectomy were caused by her thwarted maternal desires. "For me it was the end of a problem," Leigh explained. "For her, it was the end of hope."

Margie, 33 and childless, experienced a substantial sense of loss resulting from her hysterectomy. Although she had always thought that she would have children someday, it had never been the right time when Margie could have a partner, a house in the right school district, and the other things that she felt were necessary to raise a child. When she began to suffer very painful endometriosis, Margie had conducted a lot of research, taken powerful medication, done "some Native American stuff," and undergone less extensive surgery in an attempt to put off the hysterectomy her gynecologist recommended. Although she desperately wanted to have children someday, Margie finally "couldn't take the pain [of endometriosis] any more . . . just couldn't live like that." Prior to surgery she investigated freezing her eggs, but no laboratories would freeze just ovum, and she didn't have access to sperm.

Margie confided that, after hysterectomy and bs-o, "I just was *empty*." She told me that she was furious at God because she couldn't have children and asked, "Why me?" Margie explained that for a long time she didn't speak about her grief and "shoved it down . . . pushed it away." Although she was undergoing psychological therapy at the time, she never mentioned her true feelings about hysterectomy to her therapist because "it hurt too much."

In addition to becoming incapable of fulfilling her own personal longing for a child, Margie felt "nonproductive" in terms of societal expectations regarding women: "I couldn't do what I came in the world to do, supposedly . . . to have children. That's what women are here for, right? That's what society says. You know? I felt useless. I didn't feel like a woman." Later in our interview, she agonized:

> I'm not a woman. What makes a woman different from a man? Or, like it goes back to the word *female* versus *male*. I didn't feel like a woman. I couldn't have children; I couldn't do what women are here to do. I couldn't reproduce.

Margie believed that the end of her fertility had destroyed the core of her gender identity.

Sandelowski discovered that infertile women experience their "difference" as a "source of real anguish":

> Infertile women feel thwarted in their efforts to enter the female world and to exchange in the "currency of women." They feel

"lost out," marooned, and separated from their obviously fertile mothers, sisters, and sisters-in-law. . . . Infertile women are alienated . . . from the women who appear (to the sensitivities of infertile women) to flaunt their pregnancies, "rubbing it in" while rubbing their bellies. Infertile women experience a profound sense of Otherness, of being neither female nor male, infused with feelings of fascination, envy, persecution, and even rage. (1990, 34–35)

Childless respondents in my study found it stressful to pretend to share joy for pregnant co-workers, friends, and relatives. Baby showers, viewed as cultural fertility rites, were particularly difficult occasions for them. Leigh, who didn't want children, was "bored" at these events because everyone "talked about diaper rash endlessly." She complained, "What I realized very quickly on is that it is not correct to object to conversations about children. Somehow, in our society, if you *do*, then you're the bad person." For other respondents, the subject of childbearing reinforced their emotional pain and feelings of loss.

Margie complained that, when she returned to work after recovering from hysterectomy and bs-o, "everyone was getting pregnant and having children, and it sucked. I couldn't talk about it. And there was no space to say, 'It really hurts.'" There were "baby showers every other week. People puking, bringing in ultrasound pictures, talk about what are they gonna dress the nursery in." It was especially difficult for Margie to "hear women saying that they didn't want to be pregnant accidentally." She believed that she was supposed to act as if she was thrilled for her pregnant co-workers, while inside she had "ugly" feelings and really felt, "It was just gross. It wasn't OK. The things people are supposedly happiest about in the world, I hated. Childbirth, getting pregnant. Normal things . . . and there's no place for it. There was no place to say 'Geeze no, I'm really not happy for you.'" Margie avoided going to the inevitable baby showers by claiming that she was "not a party person."

No one noticed that Margie might be sensitive to conversations about pregnancy and babies until a year and a half following surgery, after she had become a substance abuser in an attempt to escape her emotional pain and ultimately resorted to stealing drugs from the hospital where she worked. After that, people told her, "We didn't know what to say. We didn't know how to ask if it was OK." While she was recovering from her addiction, Margie again felt the pain of her infertility. "I still can't look at the little clothes," she confided. "I can't buy the cutesy cards. I can't look at them." In the seven months that she had been sober before our interview, Margie had dealt with her anger through talking and writing about how it felt to be childless. She believed that she had made progress because she could now look at pregnant women and say, "Geeze, good for you."

Margie explained that directly following her hysterectomy, "I couldn't even look at children . . . but now, I baby-sat for a friend's child last week, and it was OK, it was fine. It didn't hurt to see the child." However, she is still full of remorse. When a friend recently told her she had become a grandmother, Margie "was just hysterical it hurt so much." She cried throughout our interview when talking about her inability to have a child but hoped that the passage of time would help. Since Margie is bisexual,[2] I asked her if she had ever considered having a child through a relationship with a woman who was able to give birth. Margie responded, "I think it would be harder. . . . Again, what I can't have, and I know I can't live with that. Today, now. It might be different over time."

Some of the women who were most upset about losing their ability to give birth were not necessarily those who fit "feminine" stereotypes. Gloria, 39 at the time of surgery, told me that she had always been a lesbian, that she takes after her father, and that her main source of employment is construction work. The outward appearance of this "butch"-looking woman with a blonde buzz haircut, wearing a black motorcycle jacket and chains, contrasted sharply with the grief she expressed at never having had the opportunity to become a mother.

Like Margie and other respondents, pregnant women and babies reminded Gloria of the pain of her infertility. She related that, while she was still in the hospital recovering from her hysterectomy and removal of one ovary, her teenage niece ("the little bitch") was in the same hospital giving birth to a baby whose father was imprisoned for child molestation. This provoked Gloria's anger regarding how unfair it was that she would never have children. She also complained that the hospital nurses made her exercise by walking from her room "down to the other end of the hall, and it was the cruelest thing, because the other end of the hall was the maternity ward." Gloria cried:

> And I'll never forget it; I'll never forget it. I just fell apart. . . . I thought it was so insensitive. But at that point, I didn't even know I was feeling that. I just fell apart. . . . Right now, I could cry about it. . . . It was awful. . . . I would like to have children. I can't. Yeah, it really bothers me. . . . And there were all these beautiful little babies, brand new, and me with my pole [attached to her intravenous feeding bag], and my stomach cut open, and never able to have children.

Other respondents mentioned the callousness that hospital staff sometimes displayed by not protecting post-hysterectomy women from contact with pregnant women and babies. Unbelievably, Susan told me that she was the only patient recovering from a hysterectomy in the same ward room with women who had just given birth.

However, it is impossible for women to completely isolate themselves from contact with children and babies forever. Donna told me that she baby-sits for a much younger friend who at age 23 has two children and that she does not like the way this woman treats her children. She interpreted this in the following manner:

> I would have been a good mother. It doesn't actually work out that way, but some people who are not so good parents get to have kids, and then people who might have been good parents don't get to have kids. There's a kind of unfairness to it all. And that sneaks up on me every once in a while. Like I'll be watching a TV show and all of a sudden the plot will turn to an abused child. And I get very mad at the world, that kind of thing. But I have a feeling that I still have some stuff to get out about that.

For several respondents, encounters with women who they perceived were inadequate mothers were painful reminders of the "unfairness" of their own childlessness.

Inability to Produce His Child

In addition to their own grief regarding infertility, some hysterec-tomized women fear that their male partners might leave them because they are unable to give birth to their children. According to Matthews and Matthews, "to the extent that the couple regard having children as a fulfillment of both their marriage and even their purpose on earth, infertility calls into question the meaning and purposes of both their marriage and their very existence. . . . Not only does this raise the possibility of 'responsibility and blame' being assigned to one of the partners, but the designated person may feel guilt and experience doubts about the continuing affec-tion of the other partner" (1986, 643–4). Greil (1991a and b) also found that infertile women sometimes perceived that they were unworthy of their husbands' love because they could not provide them with children. Many infertile couples are not certain whether the man, the woman, or both are responsible for the couple's child-lessness. However, when the woman has undergone hysterec-tomy, she is the obvious source of blame.

Donna, 40 years old, was relieved that her present husband, eight years younger than she is, has "been pretty good about" her inability to have children: "He was more concerned that I be healthy." Donna explained that her husband

> always had mixed feelings about having kids, so I don't think—I think it was a loss for him but not an overwhelmingly—it wasn't like one of the big goals in his life was gone. I've had friends who married childless men after they had their hysterectomy and they've had husbands leave them because of the desire to have a kid. And I sometimes have worried that he would do that some-day. But not because of anything he's said or done, you know what I'm saying? It's just my insecurity about it.

Donna's insecurity exemplifies other women who fear that the in-fertility resulting from hysterectomy renders them inadequate as wives.

Penny's first husband had already left her because she had dif-ficulty becoming pregnant, and she was later told that she was infertile from the gonorrhea she caught from her second husband. However, Penny also felt that the removal of her uterus and one ovary at age 27 "was like putting that final touch on it." She told me she "had a nervous breakdown" after the hysterectomy. At the time, she was still married to her second husband, who had a daughter from a previous marriage, and, "as far as he was concerned, he didn't make all that much money, so to support one daughter it was fine with him that he didn't have any more children." Despite the fact that he was the source of the gonorrhea that prompted her hysterectomy, Penny was grateful to this man because "he accepted me the way I was." Although he was abusive, she felt "there weren't too many men at that age, as young as we were, that would accept a woman who couldn't have children. So I kind of went with the program." Interestingly, after Penny ultimately left her second husband, she found three other husbands who didn't mind her inability to give birth to their children.

Closing the Final Door

Kessler and McKenna attempt (1978) to minimize the significance of reproductive ability as a component of feminine gender identity by claiming that females "can reproduce for only a few days each month for 30 to 40 years, which totals perhaps 3½ years over their life span when they could be identifiable as capable of reproduction." Nevertheless, I believe that these sociologists miss the importance that women feel regarding reproductive ability as a *potentiality*. Sloan, a gynecologist, maintains that "reproduction as it exists in the female self-image, even if childbirth is not wanted by the woman, remains important . . . because of the meaning it imparts as a signal of identification and totality" (1978, 603). It is the *potential* to become pregnant and carry a child that premenopausal women lose through hysterectomy—what Donna referred to as a "chapter closing." As Leigh described her co-worker who had always wanted to give birth, hysterectomy was "the final dotting of the 'i.'"

Loss of what they considered the special ability of a woman to give birth caused deep emotional grief to most of the women I interviewed. This was the case regardless of their previous child-bearing status or plans. Brooke expressed her loss this way:

> Even though I never fell into the trap identifying myself as a birthing machine, or as a mother, or as part of my identification of who I am, it turned out, six months later in my mourning process, I discovered that I am a woman who *had* the ability to give birth. Because I am a woman, I *had* the ability to give birth, and it was always a *choice*. And now the *choice* was taken away. And I was mourning that. That I no longer had the *choice*. Even though I never wanted it.

Women who had not previously considered giving birth one of their important personal goals sometimes felt remorse after they found that childbearing was no longer a possibility. Christine, childless at the time of her hysterectomy at the age of 38, commented:

> I must admit that knowing I had to have a hysterectomy made me want to have a child more than I ever wanted to before. . . . Yeah, I could always say I didn't want them now, but who knows what I might want later. And there was the *finality* that was no longer making it *my choice*. It was OK if *I chose* not to have children, but if you told me that you were going to make it so *I couldn't* have them. . . . And I certainly didn't want to have somebody else deciding it.

This feeling was present for women who already had children as well as for the childless. Even mothers who had previously decided that their families were complete found themselves yearning to have the option of future pregnancies still available to them. This confirms previous research findings that women's emotional reactions to hysterectomy are not necessarily related to the number of children they have birthed (Meikle, Brody, and Pysh 1977).

Literature on natural menopause often implies that the end of the "childbearing years" produces alternative forms of fulfillment because a woman is now free to "become pregnant with herself" (LeGuin 1976, 5). Generic use of the term "childbearing years" is problematic for women who have undergone hysterectomies, since for them the loss of childbearing potential is not a matter of chronological age.[3] Premenopausal women who undergo hysterectomy are often forced to confront the end of their fertility not only before they are "psychologically ready" but before they are "sociologically ready" as well. I have developed the term "sociologically ready" to refer to a woman's perception of life stages and where she sees herself in terms of her age cohort. If a woman's friends and relatives in her age group are still able to become pregnant, this can be very painful as a reminder of her premature loss.

Janet stated that, although she hadn't planned to have more children, before her hysterectomy and bs-o at 39, she "liked the feeling of knowing I *could* get pregnant." Janet remembers that, at her first post-surgical appointment, she saw framed photographs of a little girl on the surgeon's desk. The doctor remarked that this was his youngest daughter—"our pride and joy." Recognizing that the surgeon was at least five years older than she was, Janet resented that her ability to give birth had been terminated prematurely.

In several cases, respondents' own biological children were painful daily reminders that they would never again give birth. Novelist Lynne Sharon Schwartz describes this situation particularly well:

> How good to see your children and how good they are, scurrying around to bring you tea and chocolates and magazines [while she was recovering from hysterectomy]. Why is it that the sight of the children, which should bring you pleasure, also brings you grief? It might be that their physical presence reminds you of the place they came from, which no longer exists, at least in you. . . . Your twelve-year-old son brings you a jigsaw puzzle of a Mary Cassatt painting—a woman dressed in pale blue, holding a baby who is like a peach. It looks like a peach and would smell and taste like a peach too. At a glance you know you can never do this puzzle. It is not that you want another baby, for you do not, nor is it the knowledge that you could not have one even if you wanted it, since that is academic. Simply the whole cluster of associations—

mothers and babies, conceptions, gestation, birth—is something you do not wish to be reminded of. You seem to be an exception to the facts of life, a mutation existing outside the facts of life that apply to every other living creature. (1987, 46–8)

Yvonne told me that she and her husband never really made a final decision not to have more children, "It just sort of happened." Although her two sons were 13 and 15 years old when she underwent a hysterectomy at age 37, she had felt that "the door wasn't really shut" because her mother had given birth to four children in "two batches of two," and her husband had always wanted a daughter. In spite of her awareness that it was unlikely that she would have had more children anyway, after hysterectomy Yvonne also remembers feeling "I guess what you would call 'wounded.'" When I asked in what way she felt "wounded," Yvonne explained:

Just, I think, partly that this had happened, that I had really *crossed a bridge*. I think at that point I realized that I had *crossed a bridge*, that the womb was gone, that *the door was shut*. But I felt just wounded, helpless, wounded . . . just all over. I felt it was like you were—it wasn't that you were in a situation where you were going to die, but that you were very seriously injured in some way. Somehow you don't realize the step until it's been taken and then. . . . Yeah, that I had *closed a door, crossed over a bridge*, that was it. That my childbearing days were over. . . . Ummm, it wasn't that I was—I'm not sure that I was sad; it was just the realization that there was no going back. There was no—the little girl was not going to be around. . . . He [her husband] still says, sometimes, you know, "I wish we had had a daughter." . . . Ohhh, sometimes it makes me sad. But I realize that there's nothing that can be done about it. We just have to get along. But I think he really would have liked to have a girl. . . . Yeah, it was sort of final. . . . It was sort of that "the boys are it," more or less. The *crossing the bridge* sort of into another segment of your married life where this is it, the boys are going to grow up, and there are no more children. It's just going to be Tom and myself. . . . It was OK, but it was a realization that *a step had been taken,* really without considering—that wasn't a consideration when . . . whatever other issues were there take a back seat to this particular health issue. So it was just never brought up. And by the time it started to—when your mind starts working, it's too late already. . . . I think it's the possibility, definitely. *The possibility was being taken away.* . . . I think I just sort of accepted it. This is it, we have a nice family, we have two healthy boys, and we're happy, and this is the way it's going to be. Some people have no children.

Yvonne simultaneously felt grief about losing her ability to have another child and guilt because she believed that she did not have a right to feel that way. A common reaction by friends or relatives is to attempt to minimize a hysterectomized mother's suffering by reminding her that she already has children. Although well meaning, these reminders often prompt these women to feel that their emotional pain is unjustified. Assurances of prior motherhood completely underestimate the intensity of the emotional experience involved in losing reproductive potential at an early age, regardless of previous childbearing.

Kelly's husband had a vasectomy after their second child was born because they decided not to have more children even "if something bad happened." When Kelly found out she was going to have a hysterectomy, her husband joked, "Gee, if I'd known that . . . ," implying that he wouldn't have had the vasectomy. Kelly told me, however, that when she felt her last ovulation before her scheduled hysterectomy and bs-o:

> I had a little ceremony in my mind, that was kind of—it was a painful ovulation, but it was. . . . I had a friend who counted all the time she ovulated and she counted all the wasted babies. . . . I was sentimental about it. I liked having babies. I liked being pregnant. I liked knowing that I got pregnant. I liked planning it and saying, "Now's the time," flowers on the calendar, and knowing it was my fertile time. I was very focused on that. . . . Well, I thought about when I had gotten pregnant, it was nice knowing when I ovulated. I always had very dramatic ovulations, so it was always nice. When I wanted to get pregnant, it was nice to know that I had it.

Now that she knew she could never get pregnant again, Kelly felt sentimental about her past fecundity. Rather than the gradual and vague end to fertility that occurs with natural menopause, women like Kelly were able to pinpoint the demise of possibility. Loss of fertility potential was an issue even for women who were long past childbearing. Joyce, whose children were in their twenties by the time of her hysterectomy at age 41, and who told me she had never wanted more children, also commented that she had "a pang" thinking, "Well, this is it—you can't . . . you know, you don't have the choice anymore—*this is it.*" Deborah, who had two grown children and had already gone through natural menopause, felt more than a pang. She cried bitterly as she discussed the loss of her womb and ovaries at 65 years of age. Deborah explained that going through natural menopause had not upset her, didn't disrupt her life, "I didn't feel as disturbed by losing anything there as I did when I found out about the hysterectomy. . . . But, you see, that was like a natural process. Your menopause is a natural thing." Deborah asserted that after menopause she felt that "things are functioning the same, but this was different somehow. . . . Just something that you were no longer a woman." When I questioned her further about what she meant, she told me that she was bewildered, "Sometimes I think, 'Oh, if I could have a baby, I would' . . . but I wasn't going to have a baby at that point." Deborah struggled with the incongruity between her certain knowledge that she would never have had another child anyway, and her grief at the loss of her reproductive organs. "It was there, it was there, I really felt it," she lamented. "It was taken from me." She told me that it was hard to define what troubled her, but then suggested, "Maybe it went back to the point in time when I was afraid I might not be able to conceive [before she had children]. . . . It never occurred to me until this minute. Maybe I'll thank you for it . . . it may be important." For many women, losing the *potential* to give birth, no matter how remote, is a significant loss.

Looking Backward with Regret

Similarly to Corbin and Strauss's study of people with chronic illness (1987), I found that women who have undergone hysterectomies "engage in accounting reviews, among them a self-assessment and evaluation of past failures and successes in life, failures that can no longer be made right" (269). Respondents reevaluated past abortions, miscarriages, and even previous relationships in light of the now irrevocable fact that they could no longer give birth. Drelich and Bieber assert that "disease or surgery of any organ may be viewed as punishment for guilt-laden activities involving that organ" (1958, 330). Wendy, one of the women I interviewed, believed that her hysterectomy was a penalty for her previous sexual activity and the many abortions she had undergone. "I probably screwed myself up," Wendy confessed, "This is probably my living that has caused this."

Other respondents did not necessarily *blame* past actions for their hysterectomies, but they *reframed* previous decisions and chosen life paths that now became causes for remorse. For example, Susan believed that "I, probably of all my friends, would have most liked to have had children." After a miscarriage early in her first marriage, her doctor told Susan that if she wanted to have a family, she should do so soon because her growing fibroid tumors might make pregnancy problematic in the future. However, Susan was not yet ready to have a child because she and her husband were both busy building their careers. Later, when they had marital problems, Susan avoided getting pregnant because she believed that her situation would not be good for a child. Although she always thought she would someday have children, Susan had two abortions after her divorce because she did not want to marry the potential fathers and yet did not feel that she could raise a child on her own. She explained, "I tried to use my better judgment against my desire to be a mother and have that experience." Upon marrying her second husband, Susan made an agreement with him not to have children, and then later had a hysterectomy to remove her fibroid tumors. "The critical turning point for me, in my life, probably was that decision to stay with [first husband] instead of realizing that it wasn't to be," Susan told me. "Because then I did lose my window of opportunity to have a baby." She believes that, had she divorced her first husband earlier, she might have met and married someone with whom she could have had children. This realization came to Susan only after the hysterectomy rendered her permanently incapable of pregnancy.

The undeniable infertility that accompanied hysterectomy led some respondents to reconsider life choices they had previously made that did not conform to a more traditional feminine lifestyle. For instance, in her early twenties, Donna had felt that "there were a lot of dreams that my mother let go of, and I wanted to figure out what my dreams were before I had kids." After hysterectomy at 37, she thought that she had possibly waited too late to have children, and she regretted her previous plan. "If I'd been a 'normal' woman when I was twenty," Donna lamented, "maybe I'd have a kid now."

Sometimes insensitive friends or relatives may actually instill guilty feelings by blaming a woman's childlessness on her own past decisions or lifestyle. This happened to Terry, who was the fifth daughter in a strictly Catholic family of eight children. Her mother was a very conventional housewife who never even learned to drive a car. Terry's four older sisters also followed a traditional homemaker route. She was the first child and the only girl in her family to go to college, and she continued to earn two masters degrees, to achieve a professional career, and to travel widely. Terry commented that her sisters "never quite got me! And I never quite got them. And in many ways we were estranged through the growing up years." When she found out that she had endometriosis, Terry's first thought was:

> Holy shit! Here I am, late twenties . . . I've postponed childbearing, and although I was never interested in having a kid in my twenties, I knew at some point in my life that that was ingrained in me, that I did want to have kids. And I knew that was a threat at that point.

Even though she was not yet married, Terry tried taking infertility drugs, underwent several infertility surgeries, and attempted acupuncture, but she was unable to get pregnant. Her endometriosis actually got worse, to the point where it was destroying her gastrointestinal tract, and her gynecologist strongly recommended a hysterectomy. At that point, Terry told me:

I was psychotic. I was absolutely a mess. I think I cried for days and days and days . . . I felt like a total failure. I felt totally betrayed by my body. I felt like such a good patient, and like a "good girl," that I had always done all of what was expected, what I felt was right in my life, and somehow or other I felt like "shit, am I doing this to my body?" Because there was stuff coming out in the literature that it was only thin, motivated, high-achieving women who got endometriosis—yadda, yadda, yadda—and I thought, "If only I'd been like my sisters and if I'd only fit in, that none of this would have happened."

Rather than being supportive, her family reinforced Terry's remorse. She told me, "I remember one of my sisters saying, 'Well, if you didn't go schlepping all over the world and doing all these different things. . . . You always made fun of us for having our kids, and now nyah, nyah, we've got babies and you don't.'" Terry cried, "And it was really bad. It was a knife in my heart. It was really, really terrible." She was enraged at God but also, she said, "raged at myself that I paid a price for being different from the rest of the females in my family." For Terry, the hysterectomy confirmed her family's criticisms that she should have followed a more typical feminine gender role. She, like other women I interviewed, saw the past through the lens of the present. Unfortunately, these women could not have foreseen that they would undergo hysterectomies. Life choices that had seemed reasonable at the time were now cause for regret.

Restoring Order/Regaining Control

Learning to Live with Infertility

There is a general cultural belief that becoming a parent is within every individual's personal power. In her work on miscarriage, Shulamit Reinharz (1988, 86) maintains that "an exaggerated notion of control has been introduced into our view of reproduction" despite the reality that "both social and biological processes continue to interfere with complete individual control over reproduction." Griel (1991a,b) and Scritchfield (1989) each found that individuals often experience shock and a marked sense of loss of control when they find that they are unable to give birth to the children they expected to have at some point in their lives. According to Greil, "Because of the uncertainty of the infertility trajectory, the majority of the infertile have good reason to harbor the hope that they may still achieve the status of parenthood. They do not necessarily see themselves as permanently childless; rather they see themselves as *not yet pregnant*" (1991b, 103).

Women for whom the cause of infertility is unknown often feel pressure to keep trying new specialists and new procedures, never really reaching closure on their conditions (Becker 1994; Stolberg 1999). Respondents in my study are in the paradoxical position of having both less and more control than other infertile women: *more* control because, rather than searching endlessly for the cause of their infertility they know what the cause is, and *less* control because there is no treatment they can pursue to cure it.[4] However, hysterectomized women are at least able to mourn the definite and permanent loss of fertility and then make other choices.

Some respondents decided to adjust to a life without children. They found that, as for others who are involuntarily childless, "the transition to 'nonparenthood' usually requires major adjustments in their self-images and life plans" (Matthews and Matthews 1986, 641). Greil contends, "The normality of nonparenthood is not something learned once and for all but, rather, something continually relearned in the course of everyday life" (1991b, 52). At the time of their interviews, even many years after hysterectomy, several respondents were still struggling to adjust to "nonparenthood."

Grief regarding missed opportunities is an enduring lifetime circumstance for many women. May, who was 97 at the time of her interview and had undergone a hysterectomy at age 37, told me that, at the time, she thought her doctor had told her that she could still give birth after surgery. Although she never had children of her own, her husband had a daughter by a previous marriage. Now that May is older, she says she "made a mistake" by not allowing contact between her deceased husband and his daughter. She is resentful and jealous of other women in her residential facility whose children and grandchildren visit them, and feels that she lost the opportunity for a relationship with a step-daughter who would help care for her. Donna, only 40 years old at the time of her interview, looked toward the future and wondered "what it's going to be like to be really old and childless. . . . And you think about: you get old, and you get to enjoy your grandkids, then somebody takes care of you. So, I think that's part of—I think about that being gone too and missing from my life as well." The state of childlessness often continues as a deprivation that is expressed in different ways over the life course and that women deal with in a variety of ways. When I asked Donna if she thought she would ever resolve her grieving, she replied:

> I don't think so, no. I remember this thing with a mother of one of the Lockerbie victims [who were killed as the result of a terrorist bombing of an airplane that crashed over Lockerbie, Scotland]—they were interviewing the survivors of the people who were killed. And this mother had a plaque on her wall, and it said, 'The question is no longer how to find an answer, but how to live without one.'"

Donna felt that this quotation really "spoke to" her, and she wrote it on a piece of paper and kept it with her for quite a while. She believed that the potential children that she had lost through hysterectomy were equivalent to the children who were killed in the airplane disaster. Donna felt like a survivor who was still mourning her loss.

Restored/Reconstructed Motherhood

Charmaz describes the tendency of chronically ill people to set recovery goals in terms of "preferred identities," and their attempt to achieve "the same *sense* of self they possessed before illness" (1987, 301). Motherhood was a "preferred identity" for many respondents in my study, who often sought to reconstruct it as best they could.

Childless respondents took a variety of paths to become nurturers. For example, Susan told me, "I have seven godchildren now in my life." She commented that she takes her godchildren on "fun trips" and generally "spoils them rotten." Susan views this activity as her way of fulfilling a need to connect with the younger generation. Christine commented that she "finally got to be a mother" by taking foreign students into her home as a "host mother." Donna told me that she and her husband were considering taking in foster children. Letitia is very involved with her grandchildren and also nurtures six dogs. Brooke is presently in a relationship with a woman who has two small children who are shared with her former partner. Although Brooke explained that "I clearly will never be the mother . . . they [already] have two mothers," she is content to be "a friend, a good friend, trusted friend" to these children.

Gloria, who felt she would have made a "great mother" because "I love kids, kids love me," told me she always has other people's children around her. She has become an important adult figure in the lives of her niece and nephew, whose mother has addiction problems, and she also spends a lot of time with neighbors' children. Gloria told me she has them all to herself when she baby-sits and is thrilled that the baby crawled to her even before he ever crawled to his parents. She explained that this fulfills a need for her, "So any time kids start growing up, I always find littler ones to replace them."

Ann is in a long-term committed relationship with a younger woman. Although her partner always wanted to have a baby, Ann was at first adamantly opposed to raising a child. But, she explained, "our relationship shifted, and I went through this long crisis with my mother, with her health, and I just started thinking about things in a very different way. So, . . . I realized that I *did* want to have a child with her." Ann believes that, since she has been going through the "whole donor insemination process" with her partner for a couple of years, when her partner does become pregnant, "we'll both be pregnant in some authentic way."

Charlotte illustrated how she dealt with her infertility by getting herself "involved with children." She and her husband have always lived upstairs from her disabled sister and family. Originally, Charlotte's sister believed that she would never be able to give birth, due to her disability, although she is the one who did eventually have children, while Charlotte was the one who was unable to get pregnant. Charlotte considers her nieces and nephews like her own children and commented:

> My sister had the children—*she* wasn't *supposed* to have children and *I* was [the one who was] going to have children. And I told her, "I will share my children with you." So I found out that *I* couldn't have children, so *she* shared her children with *me*.

Charlotte has also taken in children of relatives and friends when their parents were unable to care for them and has accepted local police requests to shelter troubled teenagers rather than have them sent to juvenile hall. Charlotte is proud that all these children have grown up to be good parents themselves, and one young woman told her, "You know, auntie, I'm not a child abuser because of the time I spent with you." She continues to nurture children while working in her niece's daycare center, where I observed her gentle interaction with little ones. Thus, although not bearing the official title "mother," Charlotte, like several other respondents, has been able to live out the nurturing part of her feminine gender identity.

A few women actually did become mothers, despite their hysterectomies. Terry told me that after surgery, "I didn't feel like a woman any more. . . . My body couldn't reproduce anything. . . . I really just felt like a piece was missing. . . . I desperately, desperately at this point, now, wanted to have a kid in *any way* that I could have a kid." With great difficulty, three years after surgery, Terry and her former husband adopted a little boy, Christopher. Although she told me that "nothing can ever make up for infertility. Nothing can *ever* replace being denied that *choice*," she also commented that "adoption changed everything" for her: "Once Christopher was placed in my arms, it was as though it all melted away." She described this further:

> Oh, I felt an aura. I actually saw this sort of halo-like sort of thing. Remember those old Clairol commercials where the man and

woman run together and the world melts away? . . . I really felt otherworldly at that moment. And it wasn't just the anticipation of it. It truly was magical, and I felt this energy, and he was this little tiny, sickly kid with birth complications. And I just knew it was meant to be. It just felt so, so right.

Terry's version of becoming a mother is at least as romantic as most women's childbirth experiences. According to her, when she recently retold Christopher, now almost twelve years old, the story about "the first day I met you," he started crying, and said, "Oh, Mommy, that's so wonderful." Terry revealed to him, "It was like the tenderest moment in my life, and even though you didn't come from me, I just knew that was God's plan, that you were meant for me." Christopher just looked at her and said, "I can't imagine anybody else being my mother." Terry felt so fulfilled by motherhood that, despite a very demanding professional career and passing her fortieth birthday as a now divorced single mother, she had adopted a little girl through the Division of Social Services a few years before our interview. She told me, "I could see myself retiring and being one of those women who buys an old Victorian and fills it with kids."

Lupe, who mourned her hysterectomy because she wanted many offspring and only had two, also sees more children in her future. Her goal is to adopt several children who have no one to take care of them. "It's a cultural thing," she explained, "because we are very family oriented." When I interviewed her, Lupe and her husband were just about to start adoption classes with the Division of Social Services.

Other women do not see adoption as a viable route to motherhood. Margie, who is heartsick that she never had children, told me she didn't think that she could adopt: "I'm not rich. I'm not married. I'm not Rosie O'Donnell. Like the barriers to that are . . . I don't know if I have that energy." For many women, the female experience of pregnancy and childbirth is something they feel could never be replaced, even if they were eventually able to become mothers. Bernadette had an abortion of her only pregnancy shortly before her hysterectomy at 30. She was devastated that she would never have the opportunity to carry a child:

Well, I'm trying to be realistic here, and optimistic. That if I want to have a child, I have to—I can still use my ovaries. But that procedure, it's very expensive. It's probably going to cost me at least $20,000 just to do that. . . . I know that I can still have a kid; I just can't carry it. I have to get a good friend or relative or pay someone to do it for me. . . . I wish I could do it myself, because I wanted to go through that whole experience, you know? Gain weight, feeling it kick, and all that stuff. . . . Why me? What did I do? I don't understand this.[5]

These are questions many respondents continue to ask.

Empty Space

As described throughout this chapter, most of the women I interviewed felt a terrible *emotional* emptiness because they were no longer able to reproduce. A related issue for a number of respondents was the eerie feeling of *physical* emptiness that accompanied the removal of their sexual/reproductive organs. According to Erikson, mature women's fulfillment is founded on the fact that their "somatic design harbors an 'inner space' destined to bear the offspring of chosen men, and with it, a biological, psychological, and ethical commitment to take care of human infancy" (1968, 266). Erikson theorizes that this inner space is at the center of women's despair. "Emptiness," he writes, "is the female form of perdition," and each menstruation is "a crying to heaven in the mourning over a child," which becomes "a permanent scar in the menopause" (278). Stoller also assumes that all women have "a sense of space within." He describes this as having

> indefinite dimensions but definite significance, produced especially by the vagina and even more vaguely by the uterus, this sense being brought in time by use more clearly into the sensed body ego, in a way comparable to the building up of the infant's body ego by the felt use of the various parts of its body. (1968, 61)

These theories may be specious in their generalities regarding all women. However, it is interesting to consider whether some sense of "inner space" prompted the feeling of physical emptiness that some respondents described.

Women depicted this void in a variety of different ways. Several women used the analogy of a "hole." For example, Ethel referred matter-of-factly to "a big hole" where her uterus and ovaries had been, and Catherine described this as "a big black hole." Terry further explicated this concept:

> I really felt like there was a *black hole* inside of me. I always visualized my internal organs, and my uterus and my reproductive self as sort of ripe and juicy and fruit-like, and I clearly remember feeling like a *vacuum*, like a *black hole*, like a *nothingness* in there. It was probably one of the most devastating things in my life. . . . I felt for the first time . . . in my life felt *incomplete as a woman*.

Ordinarily, people are more accustomed to identifying symptoms of presence (e.g., pain) than absence; if an individual feels nothing, she is likely to be relieved that her body is functioning normally. However, Susan vividly described her feeling of discomfort stemming from "emptiness," which others also depicted as a physical sensation. "I remember feeling a terrible difference in my body, like there was a cavity where there hadn't been before," she complained, "It just felt *empty*."[6]

Some women claimed that the empty space created by missing organs led to physical ailments. Kelly believed that she was frequently constipated "because your bowel has so much more room to expand, it's filling up your cavity differently." Margie reasoned that when her bladder got too full it was "incredibly painful" because "it almost feels like a balloon that sinks back to where my uterus would have been or something. And like the tube is folded over on itself." Furthermore, Catherine told me that she had developed a prolapsed bladder subsequent to hysterectomy because "there's nothing in there to hold anything up. Everything is gone because of the hysterectomy." She was required to have bladder surgery after trying five pessaries,[7] which all fell out because, she explained, "There was nothing holding it in. There was *nothing* there."

Wendy speculated that the abdominal pain she felt at times was somehow related to the void where her uterus had been. She tried to figure this out:

That's what I'm wondering, if everything has shifted around. Did everything kind of go into—I think it would have to. Because so many things are long—there's so many feet of things, and cords, so if you get something that's gone, something has to go in where it was.

These respondents implied that they were missing some essential thing or things that changed the balance of their bodies after hysterectomy.

Several women were extremely curious about what would replace the empty space that their uteri had occupied. Christine had "this picture of a void but I didn't know where—I don't even know what to call it—I guess not my womb because that's your uterus, which was taken out. But there had to be some kind of closure on this thing." Barbara asked her gynecologist, "How does it fill in?" and was told, "Eventually it does take care of itself." When Andrea wondered if "that space was there, or if my organs had rearranged themselves so that the space was gone," her therapist told her he thought "that the organs had rearranged themselves." This reassured Andrea, who commented, "I felt good about that. I didn't like the thought of any *empty space* there. And I liked the idea of everybody adjusting to the new situation."

Several respondents struggled with the concept of empty space as physical evidence that they were no longer "whole women." A case in point was Letitia, mother of three grown children, who complained that after surgery, "I was no longer a woman. I was just a shell." My extended discussion with Anita regarding this issue helps clarify the gender implications connected to this image of "empty space":

INTERVIEWER: So how did you feel physically after the hysterectomy?

ANITA: *Empty.*

INTERVIEWER: Tell me about that.

ANITA: Like I didn't have *nothing.*

INTERVIEWER: Nothing, meaning?

ANITA: I was not a woman any more [begins to cry]. . . . You have to be whole to be a woman . . .

INTERVIEWER: And you feel you're not whole?

ANITA: Yup. [To her teenage daughter] Are you whole? Yeah, she's whole.

INTERVIEWER: So what do you have to have to be whole as a woman?

ANITA: All your insides back in there . . .

INTERVIEWER: But like you said, you still have "boobs and stuff."

ANITA: Yeah, but it's not the same thing.

INTERVIEWER: It isn't?

ANITA: Put it this way: I don't have anything inside me. How do these guys turn into females?

INTERVIEWER: What do you mean?

ANITA: Trans . . .

INTERVIEWER: Transsexuals?

ANITA: Yeah. What do they do, they cut off their penis and they make a hole? You know? It's like being like that.

INTERVIEWER: You think it's like being like that?

ANITA: Yeah. But knowing I had kids before . . . I'm still a woman.

INTERVIEWER: What do you think makes you still a woman?

ANITA: My kids.

INTERVIEWER: Because you have kids. What other kinds of things?

ANITA: [Long pause]. I don't know.

Anita had five biological children, and in fact had given birth to twin daughters only three months prior to her hysterectomy at age 27. Sensations of corporeal emptiness made her doubt whether she was really still a woman or was now more similar to a transsexual. Having given birth to children was the only evidence Anita believed she could produce to prove that she was still a woman. Respondents who had never given birth were unable to produce this evidence, and may feel even greater emptiness.

In fact, a few childless women made this connection. Gloria told me that after her uterus was removed:

I felt like something was missing. . . . There was a part of me that felt *empty*, and I think the part that felt *empty* was the inability to have children. It all comes back to that. I felt *empty* . . . in my stomach. Actually, although it was more in my soul than in my stomach, it was definitely physical.

For Gloria, as well as for other women, hysterectomy created both an emotional loss of childbearing ability and a physical sensation associated with the loss of her womb.

Overall, these respondents associated amputated reproductive organs with relinquishing a very valued part of their female bodies. Some respondents had even asked their surgeons to describe what the uterus looked like when it was removed, how big it was, how much it weighed. In fact, Andrea compared her womb to an actual child. She commented:

> I felt like my uterus was a child I had carried inside me as long as I could. It really became a "you couldn't save the baby" issue for me. I carried it as long as I could until it hurt me too much and I had to let it go. . . . I talked to my uterus. I told it that I was really sorry that I couldn't have kept it and I wished so much I could. . . . I'd say things like "I'm just so sorry, I wish so much that you could have stayed. I really loved you and I loved having you be a part of me. But I was sick, I was hurting and I couldn't do it anymore." A real sense of loss . . . and it did feel like I had to let it go, and I really grieved for it, as if it were a child.

George Herbert Mead speculates, "The parts of the body are quite distinguishable from the self. We can lose parts of the body without any serious invasion of the self" (1962, 136). This may be true for *some* body parts, but most women that I interviewed believed that their sexual reproductive organs were integral to their sense of self. Losing body parts associated with fertility and birth threatened their feelings of wholeness *as women*.

Recent research indicates that gynecological surgeons may currently take fertility issues into consideration when determining whether a woman undergoes hysterectomy or an alternative treatment option. However, these decisions are generally made with regard to objective criteria such as age, number of children, and sexual orientation. Preservation of fertility may be considered less important for women who are older, who already have children, or who are not heterosexual. My research indicates that these objective criteria do not always predict which women will be most emotionally affected by the loss of their wombs. Furthermore, the extent to which infertility threatens an individual woman's gender identity may not be apparent until after she has already undergone surgery.

6

"Feel Like a Woman"?

Sexuality and Gender Identity

It is clear that sexual satisfaction serves to establish and maintain one's gender identity.

—*Robert Stoller*, Sex and Gender

"Man, I feel like a woman!"

—*Shania Twain and Robert John Lange, "Man! I Feel Like a Woman!"*

MANY SOCIOLOGISTS agree that gender identity and sexuality are deeply interconnected and that sexuality, like gender, is socially constructed (see Snitow, Stansell, and Thompson 1983). As Schneider and Gould remark, "sexuality is a social phenomenon, an activity charged with social meaning. Social actors possess genitals, rather than the other way around" (1987, 123).

Sociologists are not alone in recognizing the social importance of sexuality. With regard to the effect of gynecological surgery on sexuality, Sloan, a gynecologist, reached the conclusion that: "if we are to look at the mating behavior of an animal—the human animal—as only biologic, then organ loss perhaps takes on a less important meaning. But if sexual and interpersonal dealings are beyond that, then organ loss takes on a more vital meaning" (1978, 603). This implies that the effects of gynecological surgery on sexuality are not just physical; they are mediated through social interpretation. The ability to feel sexually attractive is an important component of self-identification for many contemporary women, as is the ability to feel sexual desire and erotic pleasure. This describes the performance of self as both sexual object and sexual subject, which is the focus of this chapter.

A number of medical researchers have sought to determine the relationship between hysterectomy and sexuality. In fact, the preponderance of studies on hysterectomy focus on this aspect of surgery, and reviews of previous research (Bachmann 1990; Bernhard 1986) found wide disparities in outcomes. While some research concludes that women suffer the loss of sexual desire and the ability to enjoy sexual relations following hysterectomy, other studies find that the reverse is true, and still others report no changes. Most previous research on the relationship between hysterectomy and sexuality is based on statistical data regarding women's reports about sexual activity. This chapter focuses on respondents' subjective perceptions about their sexuality and how they relate this to gender identity.

Woman as Sexual Object

Importance of Sexual Attractiveness

Money and Ehrhardt (1972) assume that sexual fantasies are biologically driven, while Fried (1977) contends that sexual fantasies are culturally determined. Regardless of their origin, these writers agree on the typical form these fantasies take in American culture: passive female and active male. Men objectify women as the aim of their sexual desires, whereas women identify with these objects of male desire. Since men are expected to be the aggressors, women must attract their attention (see Howard and Hollander 1997).

Current American cultural norms suggest that recognition through sexual desire is an important component of women's gender identity. Furthermore, strict standards define which women are considered deserving of desire. As articulated by the Boston Women's Health Book Collective, "Society shapes and limits our experiences of sexuality. We learn, for instance, that if our looks don't conform to the ideal—if we are fat, old or disabled—then we have no right to be sexual" (1992, 205).

Anxiety regarding sexual attractiveness is created through social pressure, which requires that sexual objects must be as close to cultural ideals of physical perfection as possible (Galler 1984; Schneider and Gould 1987). This may be problematic for women who have undergone gynecological surgery and thus can no longer be considered physically perfect. Respondents understood this. Faye commented that, because of "the way men see women portrayed in the media," they focus on women as "possessions and things, and not on the basis of what's in their heads but how they look and what their bodies are like." Therefore, she believed, some men might feel, "If you've had a hysterectomy, maybe I don't want to have anything to do with you sexually because you're not the woman I once knew."

Several previous research studies focus on women's actual or perceived impaired attractiveness as sexual objects following hysterectomy (Barker 1968; Newton and Baron 1976; Hawkinson 1959; Melody 1962; Sloan 1978).Drelich and Bieber found that "for some [hysterectomy] patients sex was not only the fulfillment of biologic drive, but also one avenue for effecting human contact and relatedness. For these women, hysterectomy, with anticipated impairment of sexual functioning, threatened serious disturbances in relatedness to spouse and other men, including fears of rejection and isolation" (1958, 326).

I interviewed four women who identified as lesbian, two who described themselves as bisexual, and thirty-eight who said they were heterosexual. Respondents who expressed fear regarding diminished value as a sexual object were primarily heterosexual women. Several of these latter respondents believed that recognition through male desire played an important part in solidifying their female identities. For example, Deborah told me that, while she never considered herself a woman who "turned on the charms," after hysterectomy and bs-o at age 65, she wondered, "If I want to use these wiles, now maybe I can't." Most lesbian and bisexual respondents were not concerned about their potential loss of sexual attractiveness. For example, Andrea, who identifies as bisexual, told me:

> I suspect that being not strictly hetero accounts for my complete lack of concern. . . . I guess I was conscious that a number of "issues" defined by the medical community were products of male-defined heterosexual crap about women's bodies.

Respondents who were anxious about remaining sexually attractive referred to standards that they now felt were problematic for them. These standards included maintaining a youthful appearance, a slim figure, and physical flawlessness. I discuss each of these below. Furthermore, I describe how some women discovered that just the fact of having had a hysterectomy "spoiled" their identities as appropriate sexual objects (Goffman 1963).

Youthful Appearance

If menarche represents the sexualization of young women's bodies, menopause may symbolize the de-sexualization of mature women's bodies. Many authors have discussed the tendency to see postmenopausal women as sexless.[1] A primary reason that Joyce was relieved that her ovaries were not removed at the time of her hysterectomy at age 41 was that she believed that she had been able to postpone menopause for ten years. She commented, "I—I guess I'm *glad* about that because I was told that . . . if y-you're not producing estrogen—your face is gonna dry up and things like that." Joyce had been in a serious relationship with a younger man for several years, and she did not like his initial reaction to her menopause, which she felt was, "Oh my god, she's gonna dry-up like a *prune*!!" She explained, "Well, that's what, that's what men feel, 'cause there was this *look* on his face initially." Joyce felt that it was particularly important following her hysterectomy that she assure this younger man that she wasn't going to "age right before his eyes."

Slim Figure

Some research studies (e.g., Newton and Baron 1976) document significant weight gain following hysterectomy, while others (e.g.,

Coppen and Bishop 1981) dispute this. Several respondents mentioned that their figures had changed for the worse. Yvonne complained that after her hysterectomy she gained weight and that her abdominal muscles "never went back to where they were." She claimed that she now has a stomach that sticks out, that "I can't get rid of no matter what I do," including doing exercises and wearing a girdle, she says. Regardless of whether or not they suffered weight gain, a protruding stomach, known as a "Buddha belly," was a common complaint of respondents. Deborah told me that she had always been proud of her flat stomach, but since her hysterectomy her stomach sticks out, despite the fact that she weighs only 115 pounds. Deborah attributes this problem to the muscles that were cut during surgery. Joyce was also distressed about her figure following surgery:

> I felt that nothing *fit*! I thought that after having surgery, and, taking these two major things [the fibroids] out of my body, that my body would be thinner, or whatever. . . . I, ah, thought that I probably wouldn't have to deal with that, but, um, I felt that right afterwards for a long time . . . probably because there was swelling, or whatever . . . *nothing* fit! It was *very* aggravating!!

Christine was surprised to find that after hysterectomy

> they took all this stuff out, and I still had this belly hanging there. And I still looked four months pregnant; I think I thought it was going to go down. And it took a while to get that down, and I never got my stomach muscles back. . . . It took a while to feel confident about my sexuality.

Several women mentioned, only half joking, that they regretted not asking their surgeons to perform a "tummy tuck" during gynecological surgery.

Physical Flawlessness

As Charmaz notes, "Having a visibly altered body provides the experiencing person, as well as family and friends, with immediate images of change" (1999b, 101). These changes can be viewed as positive or negative. Because nineteenth-century surgeons claimed that gynecological surgery made women *more* sexually attractive, some Victorian women bragged that their surgical scars were "as pretty as the dimple in the cheek of sweet sixteen" (Barker-Benfield 1976, 41). Visible abdominal scars after hysterectomy bear a different symbolic meaning in contemporary American culture.

Hysterectomies can be performed either abdominally or vaginally. Since abdominal surgery is more common in the United States, most respondents in my study experienced abdominal surgery. In addition to quicker recovery, vaginal approaches are less likely to leave external scars. With abdominal surgery, there is still a choice of scars, however. Most women prefer a "bikini cut," an incision that is only six to eight inches and is nearly hidden by the pubic hairline. The other alternative is a vertical incision, which usually extends from the navel to the pubic area, and is much more visible. The very use of the term "bikini cut" implies the interest in retaining sexual attractiveness. Some women were oblivious as to whether their bodies were noticeably scarred after surgery. Susan, for example, told me, "I didn't like having a scar there, but it's not like I wear bikinis. I'm not flaunting this gorgeous body." For others it was a more important concern, symbolically, as well as materially.

Christine had undergone an abdominal hysterectomy because her benign fibroid tumors were too large for the vaginal surgery she preferred. When I questioned her about the kind of cut her surgeon made, Christine responded, "The horizontal bikini cut, thank the Lord." I asked her why she was so thankful, and she told me that after her hysterectomy she had a black woman lover who had a vertical scar that formed a keloid: "And she was a beautiful woman, and she had this zipper, really bad, right through the navel." Christine suspected that a racist surgeon was responsible for the huge scar this woman sustained.

Some women were offended that their surgeons didn't seem to care how they would look after hysterectomy. Among those respondents who resented their doctors' indifference to the disfiguring aspect of surgical scars was Joyce. She believed that her gynecologist made her feel "vain" and "frivolous" because she wanted a horizontal bikini cut rather than a vertical cut for her abdominal hysterectomy. Joyce maintained that the bikini cut "goes into the line much better . . . and that's not as obvious." She made it clear to her doctor that although "at that point of my life, no, I was not going to be wearing any bikini," she also thought that the horizontal cut "folded right into, you know, your panty line, and I thought that would be a less conspicuous type of a thing." Her gynecologist told Joyce that he couldn't do the less obvious cut because of the position of her fibroids. Although she was disappointed, Joyce figured there was nothing she could do because, while the type of scar was an issue with her, "it really wasn't with him."

Sarah's surgeon admonished her, "I'm going to cut it for the best way that I can get at it, not for cosmetic reasons." Sarah, 40 at the time of her hysterectomy and bs-o, replied, "I'm not really into cosmetics, I'm not a person who wears a bikini anyway, so that's not a concern to me." However, she was distressed following surgery to find that her vertical abdominal scar was "uneven" and "lopsided," and "I have one side of my belly that is not symmetrical." Her female surgeon explained that the operating table was "slanted wrong" during her surgery, and then told her, "Oh, we can fix that with a little liposuction." Sarah was furious with this doctor regarding what she considered her "flippant attitude" toward Sarah's disfigurement.

While most women complained that their surgeons didn't pay attention to the aesthetic aspects of surgery, some women complained that their surgeons were *too* concerned with this issue. Ethel was insulted that her "arrogant" surgeon assumed that a major consideration was how noticeable her scar was: "He kept saying, 'You know, I really can't get over what a beautiful job I did.' He said, 'You could almost be a belly dancer, your scar is so minor.'" Ethel replied, "Well, you know, I'm a professional woman. I feel I can do more than a belly dancer." She explained to me, "There were other things that I would rather he had talked to me about—how it could impact my life, the fact that I wasn't taking hormones or something. I've never been vain about my looks, and the last thing I was worried about was the scar on my belly."

Several respondents mentioned that their surgeons made comments regarding their acceptability as "belly dancers" after hysterectomy. The association of belly dancing with feminine sensuality apparently makes it the ideal symbol for beliefs concerning the loss or retention of sexual appeal following surgery. Letitia, who was only 29 at the time of her hysterectomy, told me that, after complications from surgery, she had "a hundred little tiny stitches, from my waistline to my gold mine." She looked down at herself after her doctor removed her bandages and said, "I'd like to know what you did with my belly button." The doctor replied, "Uh-oh, I bet I sewed it inside." Letitia tried to make light of the situation and asked, "Well, where do I put the ruby when I go belly dancing?" The doctor commented that she would have to "tape it on." Although he told Letitia, "I tried really hard to make this as pretty as possible," she found it more difficult to joke about her appearance when her husband started cheating on her shortly after hysterectomy. Letitia told me that she developed "emotional problems" and explained: "Well, you look down at your body and you have all these angry purple scars and you have to come to grips with that . . . you don't feel the same, you are a *changed person*."

A scar, particularly an ugly one, relates to a woman's sense of wholeness after her body has been opened up during surgery. Several women told me about frightening complications that caused their abdominal scars to split open, requiring restitching and other strategies to keep their bodies whole. Some of these women—Penny, Letitia, and Stella—said that for several months or even a year after hysterectomy they made sure to carry something big (like a large handbag) in front of their abdomens because they felt that they had to protect their vulnerable insides from the outside world. For those women who fear that they are less attractive as mates following hysterectomy, abdominal scars are not simply personal reminders; they are also fugitive signs that can be read by potential sexual partners. These scars thus become "stigma symbols," which may draw attention to a "debased identity" (Goffman 1963, 43).

Heterosexual respondents' fears that men might find them less sexually attractive may be justified. While Lalos and Lalos (1996) discovered that most men believed that the quality of their sexual lives had improved following their partners' hysterectomies, several other studies confirm that men are sometimes reluctant to engage in sexual intercourse with women who have undergone hysterectomies (Bernhard 1992; Newman and Newman 1985; Roopnarinesingh and Gopeesingh 1982). A majority of men that Bernhard interviewed believed that women "have less sex appeal and are not as satisfying to their partners" (1992, 180) following hysterectomy. She reports that some men even believed that having sex with a hysterectomized woman could cause male impotence.

Both Bernhard (1992) and Daly (1976) found that African American men were much more likely than other men to be concerned with women's sexual performance following hysterectomy. African American women claimed that African American men commonly used negative terms to refer to women who had undergone gynecological surgery and that they were obsessed with the idea that engaging in sex would be different with such women. In light of previous research, it may be noteworthy that all three African American respondents (Faye, Bernadette, and Sharon) prominently mentioned possible negative reactions from men, while three of the five Latina respondents mentioned this, and the majority of European American women did not. However, I am hesitant to make any assumptions based on this small sample, and it is also important to note that several European American women did describe perceived problems with sexual attractiveness.

Greater Availability as a Sexual Object

A few respondents told me that they suffered a different type of sexual stigma following gynecological surgery. Rather than facing *rejection* as sexual partners, they found, conversely, that because they were now safe from the threat of pregnancy, they were seen as *more desirable* sexual partners. For example, when her husband informed a neighbor that Yvonne was going to have a hysterectomy, the man commented, "Tom, you'll love it," implying increased opportunities for sexual activity. I asked Wendy, who was single and 34 at the time of surgery, if she was ever concerned that a prospective sexual partner might be turned off if he knew that she had a hysterectomy. She immediately replied, "Oh, not at all. That's a guy's *dream!*" She explained that most of the men she knew thought it was great not to have to worry that she might get pregnant. However, this also created problems for her because her lover saw her as potentially promiscuous following hysterectomy and "started accusing me of sleeping with everybody after surgery." Although Anita's partner had rejected her sexually after her hysterectomy, she also found that some other men perceived her as *more* sexually attractive due to surgery. She told me, "They would always laugh and say maybe it would feel better, like a person who doesn't have any teeth, when they go down, they won't bite you!" Whether a woman was stigmatized for becoming "sexless" or "over-sexed," the common theme is that both stigmas are cultural consequences of women's perceived role as sexual objects.

Sexual Frequency as a Cause of Hysterectomy?

The cultural association of uteruses and ovaries with sexuality is apparently so strong that the sexual act itself can be associated with the impetus for hysterectomy. Ernestine told me, "Back in the dark ages, when you got married, you gave up all rights to your body." She believed that her ex-husband might have possibly caused the problems that led to her hysterectomy by "needing to prove something by having sex on a far-too-regular basis."

Ethel described how she dealt with the notion that sexual activity had provoked her hysterectomy. When she came home from the hospital after surgery, she noticed that her mother seemed angry with her husband. Ethel asked her, "Did something happen while I was in the hospital? You seem to be very upset with Donald. I don't like the way you're talking to him. What happened all of a sudden?" Her mother replied, "Well, *I* never had to have a hysterectomy." When Ethel still didn't understand what she meant, Ethel's mother could contain herself no longer and burst out, "Well, it's probably because he wanted too much sex!" Ethel explained to her mother that her hysterectomy had nothing to do with sexual activity and continued, "You know, your two sisters had hysterectomies, do you think sex was the problem for them? Are you saying that you didn't have any sex life—is that why you didn't have to have a hysterectomy?" Ethel is not certain whether her mother ever accepted what she told her or ever truly forgave her husband. However, Ethel's mother's attitude provides further evidence of the perceived association between uteruses, ovaries, and sexual activity.

Childhood Sexual Abuse and Hysterectomy

In order to gain some perspective on respondents' sexual lives after hysterectomy, I felt it was necessary to question them about previous sexual experiences. I was surprised to find that at least seven of the forty-four women told me that they had been sexually abused as children by older males, including a brother, a cousin, an uncle, stepfather, step-grandfather, and a teenage neighbor. This caused me to speculate whether sexual abuse early in life may actually cause physical problems that could result in hysterectomy. Some previous medical research has found that a history of physical or sexual abuse may create trauma, which affects the hormonal system, eventually leading to gynecological surgery (Allsworth et al. 2001; Plichta and Abraham 1996).[2]

The Boston Women's Health Book Collective (1992, 131) claims that one-fifth to one-half of American women have been sexually abused as children, most of them by an older male relative. Moreover, they state, "If you were very young when the abuse occurred, you may have scars from vaginal or anal lacerations" (141). I am unable to determine, on the basis of my limited sample, whether women who are sexually abused as children are more likely to have hysterectomies. Anita is the only respondent who hinted that this might be the case. Beginning at age 5, she was raped repeatedly by an uncle (who ended up in jail), and she said that her gynecologist told her that the cause of her hysterectomy was having sex "at too young an age." She was unable to elaborate on this.

Woman as Sexual Subject

Sexual Response

Medical authorities and women's health advocates often disagree about the effect of hysterectomy on a woman's ability to experience sexual desire and erotic pleasure. A news article that appeared in a women's publication (Franklin 1991) claims that the American College of Obstetricians and Gynecologists (ACOG) opposed including information regarding impaired sexual response in their hysterectomy education pamphlet because it might discourage women from having the surgery. "Understanding Hysterectomy," the current patient education pamphlet published by the ACOG (1992a), states:

> It is thought that the uterus may play a role in sexual functioning, so some women may notice a change in their sexual response. Since the outer genital organs and the vagina are not affected, though, a woman's sexual activity is usually not impaired and her sexual desire should not change. Many women experience an emotional reaction, usually temporary, to the loss of the uterus. If problems persist, they should be discussed with your doctor.

This somewhat confusing statement thus attributes negative changes in sexual response following hysterectomy to emotional problems rather than to surgery itself.[3]

In strong contrast to patient information distributed by medical authorities, in the most recent editions of *Our Bodies, Ourselves* (BWHBC 1992, 1998), at least half of the section on hysterectomy and oophorectomy is devoted to possible sexual problems that may result from gynecological surgery. The potential damaging effects mentioned in this self-help book include loss of uterine contractions, pain caused by a shortened vagina or scar tissue at the top of the vagina, and diminished lubrication. The video *Sudden Changes* (Costa and Dilanni n.d.), distributed by the anti-hysterectomy advocacy group Hysterectomy Education Resources and Services (HERS), presents Dr. Marcia Coleman's assertion that there is a physiological basis for sexual changes after the removal of a woman's uterus. Several other self-help sources discuss the uterus as an important factor in sexual response (e.g., Schumaker 1990; Williamson 1992). Most alarming, an article in the menopause newsletter *A Friend Indeed* (Stensrude 1996, 2) claims that women who undergo hysterectomy lose "all hope of a rewarding sex life."

Although not apparent in patient education material, some recent medical research suggests the deleterious effects of gynecological surgery as well. According to studies published in professional medical journals, hysterectomy may detract from sexual response for women who experienced strong uterine contractions during orgasm; scar tissue resulting from gynecological surgery may make heterosexual intercourse more difficult; and internal scarring or nerve damage may cause painful rather than pleasurable sensations (Allgeier and Allgeier 1991; Darling and McKoy-Smith 1993; Reinisch 1990). Other medical studies are adamant that there are no negative changes in sexual response following hysterectomy (Galyer et al. 1999; Stein 1991).

A distinction should be made between the passive ability to engage in heterosexual intercourse by simply receiving a penis and the ability to subjectively experience pleasure from that act. Some women situate female sexual response in the context of pleasing a partner. For example, Leigh told me that her sexual drive is not as strong as it was prior to her hysterectomy: "I think that I wish that my sex drive were a little bit stronger. And I think that's in relation to my relationship with my husband. I don't think that it puts anything. . . . I *know* that it doesn't put anything into jeopardy, but I know that it would probably be a little bit nicer for *him*." However, many contemporary women are concerned with their adequacy as sexual *subjects,* not just as sexual objects. According to Cutler (1988), four components of female sexuality may be affected by gynecological surgery: libido (the mental and psychological drives to engage in sexual activity); arousability (the capacity to become physically and emotionally aroused sexually); genital tissue response (including lubrication); and the capacity for orgasm.

Some researchers studying sexual response following gynecological surgery (Darling and McKoy-Smith 1993; Dennerstein, Wood, and Burrows 1977b) have found that women's experiences differ widely. I also found varied reactions. Most of the women I interviewed did not discover changes in libido, ability to become aroused, or sexual pleasure following their hysterectomies. Although several respondents did indicate negative changes in sexual desire or response post-surgery, these sexual difficulties were not necessarily the same as those mentioned in previous studies. The women I interviewed who did experience problems complained about changes in vaginal configuration, changes in orgasm, and lessening of vaginal lubrication. All of these perceived difficulties not only rendered women less satisfied by sex but also diminished their desires to engage in sexual relations.

Changes in Vaginal Configuration

Some women were particularly nervous about resuming sexual relations after surgery because they did not know what physiological changes might have occurred. For example, Joyce explained, "After surgery, sex was initially painful and, y'know, maybe you're just . . . you're just so careful . . . because you're scared . . . you've just had surgery . . . your body's different, and you are in pain initially, so you have to be *very*, very careful." Joyce was also concerned because she had to

> sign something in the doctor's office, which is in the back of your mind [nervous laugh] a little bit . . . that—that you could end up with a short vagina or something, and a couple of other things. . . . And I thought, "Oh, my goodness . . . that *this* could happen to you! That you could end-up with . . . something else!"

The "something else" that Joyce feared finding as a result of hysterectomy was a change in sexual enjoyment due to deformed genitalia. However, once she discovered that this was not the case, Joyce was able to resume her previous sexual life.

Bernadette reported that, after her hysterectomy, she felt that "you're missing something, you're lacking something that a woman should have." She confided, "I wanted to find out if it was going to change sex. So I didn't wait that long—I wanted to find out right away." Although hysterectomy patients are usually told to wait six to eight weeks after surgery to have coitus, Bernadette engaged in sexual intercourse only three weeks later with the man she had been seeing prior to hysterectomy. She commented, "I never told him, but it's different. . . . They say it shouldn't change, but it did." Bernadette elaborated:

> I asked the doctor. I did ask him, how was that going to affect sex? He said it shouldn't change it. But it has. To me, it seems—I don't know, they [surgeons] really didn't go in that way [through the vagina]. It just seems looser, more open. To me . . . because I was always very tight. And I don't feel as tight.

Although her partner swore that sex didn't feel any different to him, Bernadette wondered, "Where exactly is that thing [his penis] going?" She said she felt as though it was just going into "dead air." Since I spoke with Bernadette only four months after surgery, and her doctor told her it would take six months to heal, she was "waiting to see if it's going to change." She speculated that maybe she was still "numb."

Bernadette's feeling of vaginal "looseness" is in direct contrast with other women's feelings of "tightness." Isabella told me that, especially soon after her hysterectomy, it was difficult when her male partner was "coming into me . . . it hurt me because it was so tight." Allison, who had a hysterectomy and bs-o at 28, complained that one of the outcomes of her hysterectomy was

> vaginal ripping during intercourse. It sounds just like a virgin, but it's not very funny when it's happening. . . . I mean—at first I was

like, "Am I going crazy? Is my vagina shrinking?" Well, that isn't craziness—that really happens!

Allison attributed this problem to "raw nerves and thinned vaginal membranes caused by surgery." She investigated and found a surgeon who "developed this surgery where he takes skin from the labia and makes extra skin over that area to make it stronger. And I've heard some nurses say that they are getting good results. I'm not ready to deal with that." Allison felt that she might have corrective surgery in the future, when her teenage children were out of the house and she and her husband would have more opportunity to benefit from it.

Changes in Vaginal Lubrication

"One of the things I noticed right off," Sarah told me, "was the extreme [vaginal] dryness . . . so that intercourse was more painful." Although most respondents felt that estrogen replacement therapy (ERT) had solved possible problems with vaginal lubrication, this did not seem to help Sarah. However, she found another solution: "What I do is just use some Vaseline or something ahead of time, either my husband or I, either way. And sometimes both. It changes." Sarah told me that she was never a person who "required sex a lot anyway." Diminished lubrication simply made sex even less appealing to her. For Donna and other women, using lubricating jelly "just became part of the ritual. It wasn't a big deal after a while."

Changes in Orgasm

A few respondents found that they were no longer able to experience orgasms after hysterectomy. Isabella told me, "I figured out that sex to me is not the same . . . because I don't have the feeling that I had before. Yeah, that's what I figured out, the sex to me is not the same." Isabella explained that she formerly was the one who initiated sex with her male partner, but because she no longer enjoys sex, "Now I say I'm sick, I have a headache. Before, I never refused, now I look for excuses not to have sex." Isabella told her gynecologist that she missed feeling sexual pleasure, and her doctor suggested, "Maybe it's in your mind." Isabella protested that it was not in her mind, and she would like to find out what was causing the problem so sex could feel the way it did prior to her hysterectomy.

Hormonal Changes: Simple Hysterectomy vs. Bilateral Salpingo-Oophorectomy

The term *hormone* is derived from the Greek word *horman,* which means "to arouse, excite, to urge" (Angier 1999, 179). Several researchers claim that the hormone estrogen is essential for female sexual response (see Cutler, Garcia, and Edwards 1984; Utian 1975). A major problem with most studies regarding hysterectomy and sexuality is that they do not distinguish between women who only had simple hysterectomies and those who also had bs-o.[4] Bachmann contends that, "[while] the relationship between natural menopause and aging has created the fear in some women that premenopausal hysterectomy will result in premature loss of sexual desire, breast fullness, vaginal lubrication, and female body contour, oophorectomy and not hysterectomy may be the basis for some of these fears" (1990, 44). Unfortunately, another gap in research studies is that they have not usually taken into account the effect of hormone replacement therapy on sexuality.[5]

Although some research studies (see Bellerose 1989; Bellerose and Binik 1993; Nathorst-Boos, von Schoultz, and Carlstrom 1993) dispute the claim that that hormone therapy diminishes sexual response problems following bs-o, several women I interviewed were convinced that ERT greatly improved their sexual response. For example, Terry, who underwent a hysterectomy and bs-o at the age of 33, was not given ERT after surgery. "I had all of the sexual problems with it—that diminished libido," she lamented. "And I didn't feel like a woman any more. I had no sexual drive." Two years later Terry went to see an endocrinologist, who "went absolutely gaga and said, 'You never should have waited two years. You were way too young. You absolutely should have been on it

[ERT] at six months! Who the hell treated you?'" Terry continued to explain:

> So I went on it [ERT] and it really made a tremendous improvement in terms of, just, vaginal lubrication was one of the first things I noticed. And also a return of my libido. I really felt much more sexual. And I absolutely believe it's hormonally related. . . . Absolutely, because I always had a very strong sexual desire. I was a young woman. And then suddenly it went from day to night. It was just nothing at all. And I knew I wasn't imagining that. I knew that was physiological, what was going on. So I've been on it [ERT] ever since. And plan probably to stay on it.

Catherine, although not as young as Terry, also found an impressive sexual difference after beginning ERT. Catherine, who had a hysterectomy and bs-o, began taking hormone therapy again in her late sixties, after almost thirty years without it. When she asked about ERT, one of Catherine's previous doctors had told her, "Well, you probably don't need it at your age. . . . At your age what difference does it make?" Her new gynecologist, who was a man about her age, said, "You're young and you're very attractive. You are a bright, intelligent woman and why not. . . . You're too young not to be able to be sexually active!" Catherine commented, "I loved him for that!'" She explained that, after beginning to wear an estrogen patch:

> I have a very strong sexual drive. Very strong. I'm a very sexual person. And that's definitely since the patch. . . . When I first put it on, it's amazing. . . . I get such a shot I just want to go right out and attack someone. I mean I get this incredible surge.

Several other women also believed that ERT was the key to improved sexuality after bs-o.

The ovaries are a woman's major source of androgens as well as estrogen (see discussion in Chapters 2 and 3). A number of researchers have suggested that androgens (particularly testosterone), rather than estrogens, promote sexual appetite in women.[6] A significant finding of Bellerose's study (1989; see also Bellerose and Binik 1993) is that women taking combined estrogen and androgen therapy experienced greater frequency of sexual desire and masturbation than did women who had undergone bs-o but were not taking any hormone therapy or were only taking ERT. Conversely, research conducted by Galyer et al. (1999) and Nathorst-Boos, von Schoultz, and Carlstrom (1993) did not find this to be the case. It is still rare to include testosterone in the administration of hormone therapy for women. Only one respondent took combined estrogen and testosterone therapy, so my analysis cannot determine the effects of this hormone. However, that one woman, Andrea, did report that she believed the addition of testosterone to her hormonal therapy made her feel "more sexual."

Battle over the Cervix

Some medical studies (Kilkku and Gronroos 1982; Kilkku 1983; Kilkku et al. 1983; Zussman et al. 1981) report that preservation of the cervix during hysterectomy may result in less sexual dysfunction than when the entire uterus is removed. In conjunction with American hysterectomies the cervix (neck of the uterus) is routinely removed along with the rest of the uterus. The rationale for this procedure is to reduce the incidence of cervical cancer, although the possibility of a woman developing cervical cancer in the remaining stump is only 0.1 percent, and widespread use of the Pap test has made cervical cancer simple to detect (Kilkku and Gronroos 1982). French gynecologists commonly perform "subtotal" (also known as "partial") hysterectomies, which remove the fundus (upper portion of the uterus) but preserve the cervix (neck of the uterus) (Laurence and Weinhouse 1994). Hasson (1993), as well as Linde and Boilesen (1997) indicate that there are two different possible sites for female orgasm. They recommend that women who experience mainly vaginal or internal orgasms should be advised to undergo supravaginal hysterectomy (which leaves the cervix in place) for benign diseases. All but a few respondents in my study had undergone excision of the entire uterus.

In *The Woman Doctor's Medical Guide for Women*, Barbara Edelstein (1982, 125) asserts that sex after hysterectomy is "damn good." She claims: "Libido in the female has absolutely nothing to do with the uterus and cervix. If anything, the cervix can make intercourse painful—it's no fun having your cervix jogged when you're making love. And your uterus is nothing but a big, unresponsive blob." Most of the women I interviewed maintained that they had never felt that their cervixes had been important to sexual response. Some did consult self-help sources regarding retention of the cervix prior to hysterectomy but were advised by their surgeons that it would be medically appropriate to remove their cervixes along with the rest of their uteruses. Before her hysterectomy and bs-o at 48, Ann asked her gynecologist if she could keep her cervix because she had read in *Our Bodies, Ourselves* (BWHBC 1992) that it could be important for "sexual reasons." Her gynecologist told Ann that "as far as she was concerned, it was "the epitome of bad medical practice and that she would never leave the cervix. She wasn't even giving me that as an option. She said that it was out of the question to leave the cervix [due to the possibility of cancer]." After surgery, Ann concluded, "My sexual response is the same as it always was."

Those few women who discussed attempts to preserve their cervixes framed these struggles as battles in defense of their sexuality. I describe their stories in some detail because they are emblematic of misunderstandings and miscommunications between gynecologists and their patients regarding sexual response. Women so rarely have a voice in controlling their own sexuality that the issue of preserving the cervix can assume great importance.

Andrea told me that her biggest question before hysterectomy and bs-o at age 36 was, "Would I still be able to enjoy sex? Because the thing that scared me the most was all these stories from women who had [hysterectomy] who said, 'Well, I used to love sex, and now I don't have the desire at all.'" Although Andrea read everything she could find on the subject, she felt that she was unable to obtain the information that she needed because all the books assumed she was married and heterosexual, whereas she was unmarried and bisexual. However, Andrea did read in *Our Bodies, Our Selves* (BWHBC 1992) that the cervix plays a role in sexual pleasure for some women. Although her surgeon "really pushed" her to take out the cervix because of the risk of cervical cancer, Andrea refused, saying, "My information doesn't match your information, and I have to make a judgment call here." She felt that, after repeated arguments, her surgeon came to respect her point of view. He "bargained" with Andrea that if he did not remove her cervix, she would promise him to have a pap smear every six months and that she would also quit smoking. They have both kept their bargains. Andrea was relieved that she "saved" her sexuality by keeping her cervix, and she claimed that now "I feel like I'm in charge. . . . Like, there's nothing in the way between me and sexual pleasure, if that's what I decide I want."

For some women, just being able to discuss the issue of keeping their cervixes allowed them to feel more in control of the fundamentally uncontrollable experience of gynecological surgery. Christine told me, "One of the hardest things for me to tell him [her surgeon]—I still had only sex with men at this time—was that an important part of sex for me was my cervix." She commented that talking to her gynecologist "was worse than buying Kotex from the 15-year-old boy!" Christine did not feel comfortable "because I never had a gynecologist talk to me about sex." So she did some research in the library and mapped-out a strategy:

I told him I wanted to schedule an appointment in which I would keep all my clothes on and just talk to him for a half hour, an hour, as much time as he could spare. . . . And he agreed to that. I said, "Do you have to take all the parts out?" And he said, "I'm going to try to leave your ovaries so that you don't have surgical menopause." And I said, "What about the other parts?" And we sort of skirted around this. Finally, I said, "There are parts of my body . . ." But I finally said to him, "I'm afraid that sex won't be the same after." And he said, "Don't worry, it will be fine." And I had read, in all the books by *men,* that it *would* be the same. And in all the books by *women* that it *wouldn't* be the same. So I said to him, "I've read one book. There's a new technique where they can leave the cervix in some of the hysterectomies. Is it possible to keep my cervix?" And he said to me, "Why??" And I said, "I'm just asking if it's possible." And finally I said, "When I have an orgasm, I can feel my cervix move, and you can't tell me that sex is going to be the same for me afterwards if I don't have the feeling." I was embarrassed as hell, but this was my last chance to bring this up, you know? And he said he would look at the ultrasounds again. . . . I went to some of my women friends, and I said, "I have an embarrassing question to ask you." First, I had to find someone who had orgasms. And would admit to it. And then I said, "Do you feel your cervix is involved in this? And is that an integral part?" And I really thought I was the only one. I couldn't find anybody who thought the cervix was important. . . . I was upset. Because even though I wasn't in a marriage relationship, I had had sex with various men and had finally gotten to the point where it felt good, after I found out things like cervix and clitoris. And educated the guy about it. And I thought, "Oh, I really don't want to go back to not liking sex, and not having it."

Other women were frustrated that they never had the opportunity to discuss retaining their cervixes with their physicians. When Yvonne met with the surgeon prior to her simple hysterectomy at age 37, he assured her that surgery would not cause any sexual problems. She told me that after her hysterectomy, however:

Sexually it was fine. But I really missed my cervix. And the things that happened with my cervix, that I don't know exactly what was happening . . . during orgasm, that I took for granted . . . what can I describe it as? A melting. . . . And with no cervix, that was the thing that disappeared. . . . That's the one thing I felt angry about, because he said, "It won't affect your sex life; it won't this and that. . . ." And I feel that it did.

Although Yvonne was still able to experience orgasms, she felt "something was different," and she finally realized "that was gone forever too." While her missing cervix never affected her husband's enjoyment of sex, they discussed it, and he was angry for her. Yvonne believes that in some ways losing her cervical orgasms was even more upsetting than losing her ability to bear children, because that would have happened eventually anyway. Despite her resentment at the surgeon, Yvonne explained, "I really couldn't go back and say, 'Hey, you took my cervix!'" She felt impotent both literally and figuratively.

"Just Different"

Although most respondents did not feel that sexuality had changed for them following hysterectomy, several other women believed that sex was not worse or better but "just different." For some, this was a functional difference. Lupe said, "I don't think I've lost any of my sex drive or anything like that . . . but I feel cleaner in terms of a female kind of way . . . vaginal, you know." Other women, including Donna and Madison, felt that sexual activity was definitely not "cleaner" than it had been before their hysterectomies; in fact, they felt that it was now "messier." Donna told me, "I think the weirdest thing was that it [semen] comes back out . . . so it's a little messier now than it used to be." Madison stated:

> I felt that when I had intercourse, there was no place for the semen to go. It was sort of like messier. . . . I really think that there's less of a repository for all this liquid to go. And so it just comes out. . . . It's sort of like there wasn't enough room for it in my body, so it would sort of be out there. I mean like on the sheets.

Madison's gynecologist suggested that maybe the reason for this was not her hysterectomy but because prior to surgery she and her husband had been using condoms. Regardless of the cause, the "messiness" didn't interfere with Madison's sexual enjoyment.

Other women perceived that their post-surgical bodies felt different in a way that was difficult to describe. Novelist Lynne Sharon Schwartz discovered that after hysterectomy and bs-o, sex wasn't better or worse, just different. Her "new body," she explains,

> feels desire and it feels pleasure, only it feels them in a wholly unfamiliar way. In bed your new body is most different from your old, so different that you have the eerie sensation that another woman, a stranger, is making love to your husband while your mind, your same old mind, looks on in amazement. All your

body's nerve endings have been replaced by this strange woman's; she moves and caresses the way you used to, and the sounds of pleasure she makes are the same, only her apparatus of sensation is altogether alien. (1987, 52)

Schwartz confesses to a sexual "experiment" with a gifted former lover to "rediscover [herself], buried deep, deep in the crevices of hidden tissues and disconnected circuits" (54). The origins of the "difference" that some women feel may involve either physical or emotional adjustments, or both.

Improved Sexual Feelings

A number of research studies (Huffman 1985; Kinnick and Leners 1995; Rhodes et al. 1999; Webb and Wilson-Barnett 1983) have found that the overwhelming majority of women who had undergone hysterectomy reported that the quality of their sexual lives was the same or had improved following surgery. Several women in my study noted that they now enjoy sexual intercourse more than they had before their hysterectomies. Andrea remarked:

I was very concerned about continuing to have orgasms after surgery. Much of the literature had scared me on this issue. I was very relieved to find just two weeks after the operation that I still was very orgasmic. In fact, I found that my level of sexual desire during the recovery period was quite high, excluding the first two weeks.

Andrea told me that she could not account for why she felt *increased* sexual desire, although, unlike many of the other respondents, following gynecological surgery she both maintained her cervix and took hormone replacement therapy that included testosterone. However, some recent medical research demonstrates evidence that increased enjoyment of sexual relations may be a common response to gynecological surgery.

In order to analyze perceptions of impairment or improvement following gynecological surgery, it is crucial to understand the quality of a woman's sexual life before surgery. Unfortunately, retrospective reports raise the possibility of recall bias, whereby women may idealize (or deprecate) their prehysterectomy sexuality. Therefore, researchers from the University of Maryland Medical School deliberately included prospective material in their study. The results were published in an article in the New England Journal of Medicine article entitled "Hysterectomy and Sexual Functioning" (Rhodes et al. 1999). The conclusions of this study were apparently so sensational that summaries quickly appeared in the popular print and online media. While the *Wall Street Journal*'s more conservative headline states, "Sexual Activity Isn't Diminished by Hysterectomy, Study Finds" (Gentry 1999), a *USA Today* article is headlined "Increased Sexual Desire follows Hysterectomy" (Rubin 1999), and an AOL headline declares, "Hysterectomy Can Improve Sex Life" (Webber 1999). This indicates a progressive sensationalizing of findings regarding sexuality and gynecological surgery.

The University of Maryland study (Rhodes et al. 1999), conducted between 1992 and 1993, investigated the reactions of 1,101 women just prior to hysterectomy and then at six, twelve, eighteen, and twenty-four months afterward. It was the largest study ever undertaken on the relationship between hysterectomy and sexuality. Seventy-one percent of the women in the sample were between 35 and 49 years old, 65 percent underwent abdominal hysterectomy (rather than vaginal hysterectomy), and 56 percent also experienced oophorectomy.

Rhodes et al. (1999) found that most women engaged in sex more frequently after hysterectomy than they had before surgery and that a smaller percentage of women reported being sexually inactive than before surgery. According to this research, frequency of sexual desire also increased significantly after hysterectomy, and a majority of women with low libido prior to hysterectomy reported that this was no longer the case a year afterwards. Although some women mentioned that they had experienced painful intercourse immediately following surgery, the percentage of women experiencing pain during intercourse dropped dramatically two years after surgery. The Maryland study also found that bilateral salpingo-oophorectomy (bs-o), regardless of hormone replacement, was not associated with lack of vaginal lubrication after surgery, and most women reported that they experienced more and stronger orgasms than before hysterectomy and bs-o.

As to the reasons why women's sexual lives may have improved following surgery, the authors of the study suggest that, because the overall quality of life may improve for women following hysterectomy, sexual functioning improves along with other factors (Rhodes et al. 1999)."[7] Research by Helstrom et al. (1994) found that dysmenorrhea is the best predictor of post-hysterectomy sexuality. Women in their study not only experienced relief from pain but also found that their sex lives had improved after the removal of their "malfunctioning" uteruses. These findings are similar to an earlier study (Darling and McKoy-Smith 1993) that compared midlife women and found that the hysterectomized group experienced greater overall sexual satisfaction than did the nonhysterectomy group. Several respondents in my study also felt that their ability to experience sexual pleasure had increased due to the alleviation of gynecological problems.

A major limitation of the University of Maryland study is that the presurgery interviews took place only shortly before women's scheduled hysterectomies. Consequently, it is possible that problems associated with the conditions leading to surgery and anxiety regarding the upcoming surgery may have negatively affected their sexual functioning at that time. Rhodes et al. (1999) admit that this may have been a problem in overestimating the positive effects of hysterectomy. Another shortcoming is highlighted in a later article by Rozenman and Janssen (2000), which claims that the University of Maryland study focused on quantity rather than quality of sexual activity and that this is a general disadvantage of quantitative studies regarding sexuality. The University of Maryland researchers reply that they believe that their study was able to measure the quality, as well as the quantity of post-hysterectomy sexual response (Rhodes et al. 2000). There is some qualitative support for their findings among particular respondents in my study.

Women who had experienced gynecological problems before surgery felt great relief afterward and told me that this did contribute to their ability to enjoy sex more. For example, Barbara was one of the women who confided that her constant vaginal hemorrhaging before her hysterectomy at age 54 had interfered with sexual relations with her husband. Although she was still recovering from surgery at the time I spoke with her, she was looking forward to experiencing greater sexual pleasure now that her "problems were fixed."

Prior to her hysterectomy at 34, Brooke was curious to know how surgery would affect her sex life, but like Andrea, she found that "there were not many books written about lesbians and hysterectomies . . . there were more like chapter readings in a book on lesbian health. Or maybe in a straight book, then there might be a chapter about lesbians." Brooke was unable to locate any information that specifically addressed lesbian sex after surgery: "It was all about sex and the husband." However, "most of the books about straight women said that they were much more sexually active after a hysterectomy," so she was hopeful that the same would apply to her. "I was very happy about that, because for two years I wasn't sexually active because of all the bleeding [from her fibroid tumors]," Brooke remarked. "When you're bleeding all the time, you don't feel like being sexual." She was relieved to find that her sex life did greatly improve after surgery ended her vaginal bleeding. Furthermore, Brooke discovered an additional benefit when she began a new relationship with a premenopausal woman. "With lesbians, you always have to worry about two people monthly having their period," she explained. Brooke and her current partner are pleased that only one monthly menstrual cycle interferes with their sex life.

Page was surprised to find that, after suffering pain for many years before her hysterectomy, she was able to really enjoy sexual intercourse for the first time in her life. She explained, "It wasn't until all this [her surgery] was all over that I realized sex didn't hurt. . . . I had no idea that it didn't hurt. . . . From the day I lost my virginity, until then, it always hurt." Page told me that when friends talked about enjoying sex, she used to think, "What the hell is everybody was talking about? Everybody has to be a masochist!" After surgery, Page realized "Oh . . . this isn't so bad!"

Other women were relieved that, following surgery, they were able to have sexual intercourse without the fear of pregnancy. Although Joy had been apprehensive that after surgery she might "lose all desire for sex," she actually found that sex was "much better." She explained that after she accidentally became pregnant with her third child, she was "never able to relax the same way during sex. . . . It wasn't that I lost the desire, it was that there was always something going on in my head, that I had to be in control, afraid that I might become pregnant. And I really did not want to become pregnant." As a result, subsequent to her hysterectomy at age 35, she "was delighted sexually."

Likewise, after having four children and a hysterectomy, Ernestine said that finally, "I was not afraid to have sex. . . . I wasn't going to get pregnant. So I didn't have to worry about taking the birth control pills that made me sick." She had previously not enjoyed sex very much and simply felt that "it was part of my job." Following hysterectomy, Ernestine was at last able to leave her abusive husband, and she told me, "I could actually relax and have sex and enjoy it. . . . Yeah! Yeah! I had more sexual pleasure than I ever had, *ever!*" As Esther remarked regarding her own hysterectomy, "They took out the cradle, but not the playpen." In common with women who felt more sexual dysfunction following gynecological surgery, women who felt greater sexual enjoyment related their changed sexual experiences to both physical conditions and social circumstances.

A Post-hysterectomy Revelation Regarding Sexuality

Howard and Hollander (1997, 18) claim, "Sexuality becomes a way of expressing gender." Sexual orientation remained stable following surgery for almost all respondents. Andrea, who considered herself bisexual, retained that orientation. Margie considered herself bisexual prior to surgery but only had sex with women. Although she now has sexual relationships with male partners, she attributes this to "experimentation" that is not related to her hysterectomy. Women who identified as heterosexual prior to hysterectomy continued to identify that way, with only one exception, Christine.

Christine's story is highly unusual, but it highlights post-hysterectomy revelations regarding sexuality. Before her hysterectomy, Christine considered herself thoroughly heterosexual. Then, while still in the hospital recovering, she dreamt about rape, "but not in the sense of somebody inserting a penis, but of somebody putting in their hand and grabbing out my uterus." Christine told me that she was in pain and very angry, thinking, "This is not fair, why does this happen to me? Why does this happen to *women? Why am I a woman?*" She was particularly angry with men "for all this misinformation, that they were all the doctors, and it was very hard to find a woman doctor. I was mad at men for saying it's 'nothing.'" Christine fought with and broke up with her lover of six years, who was married and a grandfather, because she felt that he was abandoning her after surgery. She found sex with him uncomfortable and began dreaming about sex with women. Christine's psychiatrist told her that just because she had dreams about women didn't mean she was a lesbian, to which she replied, "Of course I'm not a lesbian!" Nonetheless, Christine began to find that she was attracted to women, and, at the time of her interview, fully identified as a lesbian. She attributed her change in sexual orientation directly to having undergone hysterectomy. When I asked Christine how she connected coming out as a lesbian with gynecological surgery, she told me:

> I think that—this is very nonpolitically correct. I think I didn't feel like a woman. . . . I don't think I *ever* felt like a woman, but this [the hysterectomy] made it even clearer. . . . I don't think it's normal for women to have hysterectomies at age 38. I don't think it should happen. But I think it let me face what I couldn't face before.

Notwithstanding further questioning, Christine was unable to clarify whether she meant that she had always been attracted to women but felt freer to act on this following her hysterectomy, or whether she confused sexual preference with gender identity, since gender identity is often assumed to implicate sexuality. Christine is perplexed about this herself. Her transformation to (or realization of) a lesbian identity might have taken place even without gynecological surgery, but it is significant that *she* believes that she would still be heterosexual had she not undergone hysterectomy.

A possible explanation for Christine's change in sexual orientation may be found in the distinction she discovered in the types of orgasm she was able to experience before and after surgery. Although she fought to keep her cervix, Christine's surgeon told her he was unable to preserve it, but informed her "how they sort of make a substitute out of what's left there." However, this was not an adequate solution for Christine, who complained:

> Now, I'm not really sure I understand how that was done. But they close off the opening so there is something there, but it doesn't feel the same. . . . Yeah, but I sort of had, afterwards, you know how people have phantom limb pain? I could feel it [the cervix] sometimes . . . yeah. In a positive way. Yeah, and I'm sure it's like memory and imagination. . . . Yeah. I don't [feel it] anymore. I think the memory is fading.

Although Christine claimed that she was uncertain as to the complete reason that her sexual orientation changed, she did assert that the sexual sensations that she associated with the cervix are "less involved with lesbian sex." Furthermore, her very pronounced anger toward men, whom she resented for removing women's wombs while not being vulnerable to gynecological surgery themselves, added a nonphysical component to her motive to find a differently gendered partner.

Women who underwent equivalent gynecological surgeries had diverse postsurgery experiences regarding sexual attractiveness, desire, and erotic pleasure. The effects of organ loss on sexuality were not just physical; they were mediated through social interpretation. The biological and the social are inextricably linked in human sexuality, and respondents' postsurgery experiences confirm this.

7

Biographical Work and Impression Management

Maintaining and Reclaiming Gender Identity

Unlike other kinds of work done for one's self or others, biographical work must be done by affected persons themselves. Only the person whose biography has been rendered discontinuous can put it back together again. However, others may provide assistance with that work by providing identity boosters, mitigating performance failures, and so forth.

—*Juliet Corbin and Anselm L. Strauss,*
"Accompaniments of Chronic Illness"

Most self-presentations are sincere attempts to show others who we "really are" in order to facilitate social interaction. . . . Indeed, much impression management occurs below the level of awareness and is simply an immediate, seamless adjustment to changing social situations.

—*Judith A. Howard and Jocelyn Hollander,*
Gendered Situations, Gendered Selves

SEVERAL RESPONDENTS asserted that they were not concerned about possible gender implications of gynecological surgery. For example, when discussing the removal of her ovaries and uterus, Faye declared, "I'm no less female. . . . That's not what identifies me as female." Wendy affirmed, "I never felt like I was less of a woman, ever." However, many other respondents revealed that maintaining or reclaiming their gender identities was problematic in some way. As I have demonstrated throughout previous chapters, gynecological surgery is not a uniform experience.

Other researchers, including Schneider and Conrad (1980; 1983) maintain that some medical conditions do not automatically stigmatize the sufferer; they carry "stigma potential." According to Conrad, "Several writers have suggested that although an illness like epilepsy may be potentially stigmatizing, stigmatization is not necessarily a universal experience, and may vary by a variety of factors (e.g., age of onset, family's reaction, social resources)" (1987a, 10). Scambler (1984) distinguishes between *enacted* stigma, which results from discrimination by others, and *felt* stigma, whereby individuals feel shame because they believe they deviate from some societal norm due to their condition.

While few women I interviewed experienced overt discrimination based on having undergone hysterectomy, many perceived that particular aspects of their condition held stigma potential. I describe examples of these aspects in previous chapters, including loss of "female hormones," inability to become pregnant, and changes in sexual response. Respondents who believed that their condition was potentially stigmatizing undertook *biographical work* and engaged in *impression management* as strategies to maintain or reclaim their identities as women.

Biographical Work

Comparable to other individuals who experience biographical disruption as the result of medical procedures or conditions, respondents who perceived that their previous gender identities had suffered damage often sought to "take action to retain and/or regain some degree of control over biographies rendered discontinuous" (Corbin and Strauss 1987, 251). This requires *biographical work,* which is "[work] done in the service of one's biography —including its review, maintenance, repair, and alteration" (264).

For example, as I described in Chapter 5, some respondents, no longer capable of pregnancy, sought to reclaim the nurturing aspect of their feminine identities in other ways. Terry told me that when she initially discovered that surgery had ended her "dream of motherhood":

> For the first time I really in my life felt incomplete as a woman. . . . I never felt as though my reproductive organs complimented or completed me. But the absence thereof really was devastating. I really felt castrated. I really felt neutered in many ways. . . . I never thought about them until they started giving me trouble. And I felt when they were taken from me and when I was trying to take care of them and they didn't respond and I truly lost them, that my womanhood, or a part of my womanhood, had been taken away.

Biographical work, including the adoption of two children, enabled Terry to later resolve her feeling of lost identity:

> My uterus and ovaries didn't make me who I am. Although at the time I really felt as though that defined my femininity and my womanhood . . . *but that isn't what my womanhood is all about.* It's not some tissue with hormones in it that define who I am as a human being. There's much more than that emotionally and spiritually.

Several respondents (discussed in Chapter 3) considered taking medication a means to replace their "female" hormones. Catherine, who declared, "Hooray! I'm a woman again!" was one of these women.

For some respondents, biographical work consisted of reconceptualizing what it *meant* to be a woman. Andrea explained that, directly following hysterectomy,

> it was incredibly traumatic and very surprising to me, that at some level I had bought into this biological determinism about my gender. . . . Well, I felt if I didn't have those parts and what made me female . . . I think much more about me as a physical woman than I did before. . . . It's just that having that surgery was a big wake-up call for me, that I wasn't paying attention to my physical self

and integrating that with my sense of my identity as a human being. . . . Initially, I felt really confused. What was I? If I didn't have
those parts, how could I be a woman?

Andrea undertook a period of contemplation and reassessment,
and later concluded that her surgery gave her the opportunity to
reclaim a different definition of *womanhood:*

It sort of jolted me into an awareness that I needed to create a new
paradigm for myself, that there wasn't one out there that I could
just tap into. . . . And this was a new opportunity for me to create
my *own definition of female identity,* a woman's body. And in that
process I found myself becoming very, very empowered.

Respondents who undertook biographical work believed that this
labor enabled them to reclaim their gender identities by redefin-
ing their locations within the category *woman.*

Impression Management

Presenting an Appropriate Gendered Image

Social science has long acknowledged the importance of social relationships to an individual's sense of identity (e.g., Cooley 1983;
Mead 1962). While biographical work denotes a substantial internal transformation, *impression management,* the process by which
people present particular images of themselves in front of others
(Goffman 1959), is more concerned with the socially interactive
component of stigma potential. It is therefore a more external
management strategy than is biographical work. This does not
imply that the impression people show others is necessarily inau-
thentic (Kessler and McKenna 1978). In fact, "most self-presentations are sincere attempts to show others who we 'really are'"
(Howard and Hollander 1997, 101). Moreover, repeated performance of certain identities in everyday interactions may inevitably
"ossify" into *true selves* according to Blumstein (1975). Rosenhand
discovered that, following hysterectomy, feelings of femininity for
many women were influenced by "outside reaction, confirmation, and interaction" (1984, 50). This was the case for most re-

spondents in my study. While not all of them undertook biographical work, most of them practiced impression management in order to portray themselves as feminine, and therefore female.

Passing

Goffman (1963) distinguishes between *discredited* stigma, which is physically obvious to others, and *discreditable* stigma, which may be hidden because it is not visible to others. Whereas individuals with discredited stigma must save face in social encounters, those with discreditable stigma must control information in order to "pass" as *normals*. *Passing* refers to "the management of undisclosed discrediting information about self" (42). Although not all respondents viewed gynecological surgery as discredited stigma, many of them perceived that it was a discreditable stigma. As is common in the case of discreditable stigma, according to Goffman, these women employed information control to deflect the possibility of becoming discredited through social knowledge of their missing sexual reproductive organs.

Gender is attributed to social actors through the recognition of cultural cues, and passing is enabled both by the person who displays these clues and by the observer who interprets them (Kessler and McKenna 1978). Garfinkel (1967) contends that the strategies used by transsexuals and transvestites to impersonate women are the same as those that "real" women use to construct and maintain their gender identities, and Susan Brownmiller asserts that "women are all female impersonators to some degree" (1984, 175; see also Bartky 1998; Bordo 1993). Passing as a woman involves using culturally accepted norms of appearance and behavior. These "gender displays," rather than indicating *natural* differences between males and females, demonstrate how competent an individual is at performing a culturally prescribed gender role (Goffman 1976). Respondents had an important advantage over transsexuals and transvestites in performing feminine identity because they had been socialized from birth in this gender role.

According to Kessler and McKenna, since gender is a social fact, an individual's gender identity can be seen as "the same as the gender attribution which is made about them," and "public physical appearance" is a major aspect of initial gender attribution (1978, 39). Furthermore, they explain:

> Although internal organs are important *biological* criteria for the attribution of gender (the individual who can produce and ejaculate sperm is male, the individual who can produce an egg and nourish a fetus is female), in everyday life it is obvious that we do not decide whether someone is female or male by determining whether they have ovaries or testes, a uterus or sperm ducts. We assume, once we make a gender attribution, that a person has the appropriate internal organs, but should we find out that they do not (e.g., we might discover that someone has had a hysterectomy), we do not change our attribution. . . . Attributions, once made, are extremely resistant to change, and information about the person is fitted to the attribution, rather than vice versa. (56)

If an individual's discreditable stigma relates to body parts that everyone is expected to conceal in public, passing is inevitable. Like other people who lack certain hidden body parts, respondents "conceal their unconventional secrets because of everyone's having to conceal the conventional ones" (Goffman 1963, 75). By manipulating social aspects of gender, respondents were thus able to create and reinforce public perceptions that they had biologically female bodies.

Like the transsexual Agnes, who attempted to be "120 percent female" (Garfinkel 1967, 129), several women aspired to demonstrate to others that they were undoubtedly very feminine, and therefore still female. Some respondents even believed that they had to be "accountable" as women immediately after hysterectomy. A case in point is Joyce, who told me:

> My feeling was basically . . . that I wanted to portray myself as, when people came to see me, that I was really OK . . . and . . . I really wanted people to see that I was OK. Because, well, at that point, people weren't having, well, people had had that surgery, but none of my friends had. So, I think it's . . . really important . . . I tried to put on a . . . sounds ridiculous, but, just make, have myself look as best as I could, with a pretty nightie, pretty robe,

and, you know . . . if somebody's coming for a short visit, let them see me in the best possible light, that I was really OK with it, and I wanted people to know that I was OK . . . people treat you the way they see you . . . and I definitely wanted to portray that . . . I didn't want anybody having the feeling, oh, poor me, because . . . I was gonna get back into my life as soon as I possibly could.

Implicit in Joyce's discussion of wearing a "pretty nightie" and a "pretty robe" is the concept that getting "back into her life" meant reassuming her feminine identity.

Several of the women I interviewed mentioned employing *disidentifiers*, which are symbols used to distract observers from discovering potential stigmas (Goffman 1963). Following gynecological surgery, these women deliberately did certain things—like growing longer hair, using more makeup, or wearing sexier lingerie—which they believed would make them look, and therefore feel, more feminine. For example, when Ethel's female cousin visited her about two weeks after surgery, Ethel was in a nightgown and robe and feeling sorry for herself: "And I remember I had long hair and I hadn't done anything much with it except wash it, and she put a pretty band around my hair, and she [her cousin] teased it a little bit and she said, 'You put on some makeup!'" Ethel identified this feminine "fixing-up" as an important step toward regaining her sense of self following hysterectomy. Bartky claims that "to have a body felt to be 'feminine'—a body socially constructed through the appropriate practices [she refers specifically to beauty regimes]—is in most cases crucial to a woman's sense of herself as female" (1998, 39). There is a common cultural assumption that men have to prove their manhood but women can take their womanhood for granted. In reality, substantiating femininity is a never-ending task for most women, since stringent cultural norms guarantee that they will always be insecure as to whether they are "woman enough." This insecurity regarding feminine appearance was a particular concern for heterosexual respondents following surgery.

The way in which respondents employed impression management is further demonstrated by Sunny, who said, "Before my hysterectomy, I certainly equated womanhood with the birthing thing." However, following surgery she perceived that gender identity had become tied to her ability to present herself as "an attractive woman" and that presenting herself that way was crucial to her professional success. "Well," she explained,

> There are certainly times when I decide I'm going to dress one way more than the other, depending on what I want to represent that day. Or will I need to manipulate something more that day? So, if I'm going into a meeting with a lot of obnoxious men, and I need to get something my way, I may dress in a way that I think will get me more of what I want. . . . I would definitely use it to my advantage. . . . You know, I would put together a presentation that I thought was going to help me get what I need to get. . . . And if they're paying attention to my femaleness by listening to what I have to say, and that's what I have to do, that's fine with me. . . . And so, it's absolutely about manipulating the situation to suit yourself.

Sunny revealed that creating an attractive feminine appearance involves a tremendous amount of work, and she also admitted that it seems "more crucial" to her "feelings of self-confidence" since her hysterectomy and bs-o. In general, respondents' contentions that they were still women were strongly reinforced by other peoples' perceptions of them as women.

Information Control

Respondents who perceived that having undergone gynecological surgery was a discreditable stigma most frequently mentioned the need to control information in connection with potential heterosexual partners. Isabella, 39 years old, described a classic example of managing possibly stigmatizing information. At the time of our interview, Isabella was still involved with the same man that she had been with at the time of her hysterectomy two years earlier. Isabella confided that if she lost this lover, she would conceal the details of her surgery from other potential male partners "because the man have a taboo because the woman is a woman if they have orgasm and everything. When the woman takes out these parts, she isn't a woman . . . they say sex isn't the same." Isabella was afraid that if she did find a new boyfriend, "Maybe sooner or later they would find out [that she had a hysterectomy and bs-o], when I don't have my periods," and she would be rejected. In fact, Isabella told me that, besides her family, her boyfriend, and her doctors, I was the only person she had ever told that she had a hysterectomy.

Gramling and Forsythe (1987) contend that an individual sometimes chooses to reveal a stigma in order to gain special consideration or to admit to the lesser of two stigmas. This relates to Charmaz's (1991) distinction between *informing* and *disclosing*. She defines *informing* as telling with an objective. However, regardless of the objective, there is still a risk in informing anyone, because it is never certain how far the revelation will spread (Goffman 1963).

Bernadette's situation presents an example of the inherent dangers connected to informing. Bernadette, 30 years old, was in nursing school, and following her hysterectomy, she was tired, in pain, and depressed. Although at first she was "embarrassed" to tell her supervisor about her surgery, Bernadette felt that she *had to* in order to explain why she wasn't performing her best work. While she believed that it was crucial to inform her supervisor, Bernadette was afraid that this woman would tell other people, who she felt might then look at her "differently." Bernadette complained, "Like, there is this guy in there who likes me, and if she ever tells him, the guy wants to date me and this and that, and I'm like, 'Oh, god . . .' I don't want him to know, just in case I might want to date him." When I asked Bernadette to explain, she told me, "He might not understand all the—he might not know what that [hysterectomy] means. He might think I don't have any. . . ." When I asked if she meant he might think that she didn't have any *vagina*, she said, "Right." Bernadette thus faced several dilemmas. Informing her supervisor meant that potentially discrediting information might spread; she might be rejected by a possible boyfriend on the basis of incorrect assumptions regarding her condition; but she could not explain the reality of her condition to this man without informing him of her already potentially discrediting stigma.

The greatest difficulty in bearing a discreditable stigma can lie in determining whether "to display or not to display; to tell or not to tell; to let on or not to let on; to lie or not to lie; and in each case, to whom, how, when, and where" (Goffman 1963, 42). Accordingly, many respondents in my study agonized over whether to reveal their gynecological surgeries, particularly to new or potential lovers. Several other studies indicate that women often do not inform male partners that they have undergone gynecological surgery due to fear that men will leave them.[1] Since Bernadette is Black, it is interesting to note again (as discussed in Chapter 6) that previous research found Black women particularly concerned with concealing information from male partners because they perceived that Black men held negative attitudes toward women who had undergone hysterectomy. Furthermore, since these women also believed that men were not really capable of discerning the difference, a number of them admitted that they would not inform potential partners that they had undergone gynecological surgery (Richter et al. 2000). Despite this emphasis in the literature on Black women's concealment, Latina and European American women I interviewed also confessed to nondisclosure.

Although it is fairly easy for women to hide the fact that they have undergone hysterectomies, *felt stigma* can be prompted by discoveries made while passing. Goffman noted that an individual "who passes leaves himself [sic] open to learning what others 'really' think of persons of his [sic] kind, both when they do not know they are dealing with someone of his [sic] kind and when they start out not knowing but learn part way through the encounter and sharply veer to another course" (1963, 84).

This happened to Janet when a man she had just started dating thought he was complimenting her by telling her how great she looked for a woman over forty. She asked him what he meant, and he explained that many women her age had "dried-up skin and wrinkles" because they had undergone hysterectomies. When Janet revealed that *she* had in fact experienced this surgery, the situation was embarrassing for both of them because it unexpectedly revealed a previously hidden stigma.

The Role of Intimate Partners

"Implications for the Self"

The quality of their relationships with intimate partners was the most significant factor in respondents' stated abilities to maintain or reclaim their gender identities following surgery. Sustained intimate relationships are particularly important to identity because "the opinions of those people who matter most to us—whose opinion we care about greatly . . . have a stronger effect on our self-concepts than the views of those to whom we are indifferent" (Rosenberg 1981, 598). Furthermore, "identities that are enacted in intimate relationships should have important implications for the self" (Blumstein 1975, 308).

With specific regard to gynecological surgery, Darling and McKoy-Smith (1993) emphasize that "on the surface a hysterectomy may appear to be a biological event for a woman, but it is also a psychological event for the woman, couple, and family, which can result in both sexual and relational changes." Previous research indicates that husbands' or male partners' reactions to women's hysterectomies are important in determining women's emotional recovery following gynecological surgery.[2] Unfortunately, most researchers who have studied the role of relationships in recovery from hysterectomy have failed to recognize that women's intimate partners might include women as well as, or instead of, men. Regardless of whether they were heterosexual, lesbian, or bisexual, respondents' ongoing relationships were crucial to their subjective feelings of gender identity. Since intimate partners can potentially support, ignore, or undermine biographical work and impression management strategies, women encountered widely varying experiences.

Supportive Partners

Goffman (1963, 97) indicates that intimate partners can serve as a "protective circle," and Charmaz (1983, 181) finds that cooperation from an intimate partner is essential "to restore a floundering prior self." Furthermore, while Corbin and Strauss claim that "only the person whose biography has been rendered discontinuous can put it back together again," she also asserts that "others may provide assistance with that work by providing identity boosters, mitigating performance failures, and so forth" (1987, 264).

A number of respondents discovered that supportive partners helped them to sustain or recover their sense of themselves as whole women. One example is Andrea, who identified as bisexual, and was in a relationship with a "nontraditional male"[3] at the time of her hysterectomy. Andrea believed that "having a partner whose gender identity did not fit heterosexually defined norms" was a particularly important factor in her recovery:

> All of these experiences [after hysterectomy] were happening in a context of my awareness of *my body* and *my needs*, not in the context of a duo where I had to fit my needs with those of my male partner. In other words, I acted like a lesbian and expected my partner to respond as a lesbian feminist would, and he did. So I was very happy. I think my bisexuality clarified my feminism to focus on *me*, and *my womanhood*, in a way that even feminist heterosexuals have trouble achieving. Excluding men from your world for ten years tends to do that. I have very high expectations of the men in my life. Very few meet them. I was really lucky during my surgery. . . . I made it very clear to [my partner] that his role was to please me in whatever way he could. His feelings about that were the same as mine, and he felt just as strongly about it as I did. His role in our relationship was to support me physically, emotionally, sexually, intellectually in any way he or I could think of, as I was the needy one at the time . . . one of the rewards for having a partner whose gender identity did not fit heterosexually defined norms.

Brooke also believed that having a nontraditional partner was an important factor in her adjustment. At the time of her hysterectomy, she was in a relationship with an older woman who was "always there, very caring." This partner accompanied Brooke to all of her doctor's appointments and helped her to make decisions regarding surgery. In addition, since her partner was in the midst of natural menopause, Brooke felt she was particularly effective in communicating that lack of menstruation did not mean loss of womanhood. Brooke considers her current partner particularly supportive as well; she encouraged Brooke to participate in our interview as a means of working through her feelings about hysterectomy. In fact, all four lesbian respondents reported positive post-hysterectomy experiences with their female partners. Research conducted by Richter and Galvotti (2000) and Lees, Shelton, and Groff (2001) confirms this potentially supportive aspect of lesbian relationships.

Many heterosexual women in my study also received important support from their partners. These men were crucial to assuring hysterectomized women that gynecological surgery had not significantly changed who they were. For example, Charlotte beamed as she commented about her husband: "That man loves me for what I am!" Ethel confided, "I have the kind of husband who makes you feel good all the time." Several male partners offered tangible as well as emotional support. For instance, Donna's husband never left her side because he knew she was upset after her hysterectomy. "He stayed at the hospital for the entire time; he slept on the sofa," she reported. Susan told me that she and her partner planned their wedding so that it would take place before her hysterectomy, and that they scheduled her surgery during semester break because he was a college professor and could take better care of her at that time. Susan described him as "a very kind and loving person." The very fact that he continued with plans for their wedding while knowing that she was about to undergo gynecological surgery emphasized to Susan that he still saw her as a female mate.

In addition to providing emotional and material support, several male partners explicitly affirmed that they considered respondents to be complete as women, despite missing organs. When I asked Sunny if she ever sensed that her husband's feelings about her had changed following her hysterectomy and bs-o, she replied,

> I had no feeling that that was the case. I don't know if this matters, but Steven is just a very accepting, loving person. Steven is not a person who tells me that he doesn't like my hair, or he doesn't like my clothing. He just loves it. So *whether I had a uterus or I didn't have a uterus,* or whether I had the biggest breasts in the world or whether I didn't . . . if I gained fifty pounds, he would still love me. So I think I was very fortunate that I never experienced any of that [rejection] because of the person that he is.

Similarly, Sarah commented that her husband was "wonderfully supportive":

> Ummm, his comments and his support were never oriented toward my *female organs,* or specifically toward the operation. He was so glad to have *me* back. If that hadn't been there, I think it would have been very different. But he never made that a stumbling block in our relationship or our sexual life. He was always there, and I never questioned that loyalty and that support. And I would say in retrospect, that was probably why I hung on, because I had that support. Yeah, I think that was all the difference in the world.

For several other women, support from intimate partners also made "all the difference in the world" in their efforts to maintain or reclaim gender identity following gynecological surgery.

Fear of Rejection

A study conducted by Bernhard, Harris, and Caroline (1997) found that, although couples initially reported that they communicated thoroughly about the woman's hysterectomy, additional probing revealed that they had actually communicated very little. Many women that I interviewed admitted that they had not discussed with their partners their true apprehensions regarding the possible detrimental gender effects of gynecological surgery. Several respondents feared that revealing their own insecurities could destroy their relationships because disclosure might initiate their partners' doubts. These women often made certain that their husbands or boyfriends were away from home or in another part of the house, out of earshot, at the time of our interviews.

Respondents who were not candid with their partners were not able to fully reap the benefits of support because they were more concerned with protecting themselves from possible negative reactions. Darling and McKoy-Smith (1993) report that many women fear rejection following hysterectomy, particularly when they sense that their male partners are unconcerned about their feelings or believe that they have lost sexual attractiveness. This corroborates finding by other researchers (Ananth 1983; Dennerstein, Wood, and Burrows 1977a; Roeske 1978).

Respondents may be somewhat justified in fearing rejection. Bernhard (1992) found that although men were fairly ignorant about the effects of hysterectomy, they perceived generally negative psychological, social, and sexual outcomes. She discovered that serious relationship problems might result from societal and medical assumptions that the uterus is "the central and most important aspect of a woman's femininity." A few men she interviewed even stated that they would leave a woman who had a hysterectomy because that might make them feel less "virile" or "manly." Bernhard refers to Wolf's findings (1970) that many men believed that their own sexual identities could be threatened by hysterectomy because, without their uteruses, their wives were no longer women. In Bernhard's study, although men whose partners had undergone hysterectomy did not believe that surgery had affected their *own* partner relationships, several of them claimed to know couples who had divorced due to the women's hysterectomies. Other studies demonstrate that, while some men might not physically leave women who have undergone gynecological surgery, they may leave them emotionally or sexually (Newman and Newman 1985; Roopnarinesingh and Gopeesingh 1982).

Rejecting Partners

Charmaz emphasizes that the occurrence of medical conditions can be detrimental to intimate relationships. She cautions: "Perhaps the most telling moments and dramatic turning points occur in interaction with others. Ill people can find themselves being betrayed, stigmatized, exploited, and demeaned. . . . Shock follows such an incident since the nasty surprise uproots one's taken-for-granted assumptions about oneself, relationships, and social location" (1994, 235). Since social perceptions of uteruses and ovaries so strongly involve issues of sexuality (as discussed in the previous chapter), women who undergo gynecological surgery may be particularly susceptible to negative reactions from intimate partners.

Several women I interviewed found that partner relationships were destructive to their attempts to maintain or reclaim their gender identities following surgery. Although some men were not as helpful as respondents would have liked them to be, "didn't do enough," or "didn't get it," a few men were outright rejecting, causing emotional harm.

Anita was particularly unfortunate in her choice of partner. At the time of her hysterectomy at 27, she was living with the father of twins she had given birth to three months earlier. He informed her that he wanted to break off their relationship because sex "might feel funny because there was nothing there." Anita recognized that her partner meant that "nothing there" referred to the absence of her uterus. Her partner's attitude hurt her deeply, particularly when he justified "going out, getting it [sex] someplace else" by telling her that she was "not really a woman anymore." This not only led to the breakup of that relationship but also initiated Anita's own doubts regarding her womanhood. She told me that she began to fear, "Maybe he was right; maybe I'm *not* a woman anymore."

Letitia claimed that her husband acted as though her hysterectomy and bs-o were "a direct attack on him." Since he believed that she "had lost her womanhood," he perceived her surgery as an "assault on his masculinity." Letitia told me that, following surgery, "he accused me daily of being a lesbian, the whole bit." Although she found out that her husband was "seeing other women," Letitia didn't blame him because she felt "guilty" that after surgery she was "no longer the woman he had married." Due to her husband's rejection, Letitia came to believe that "my life was ruined, and I was not worth anything, and on and on. . . . I felt useless and ugly and that I was *no longer a woman*. . . . Before surgery I was a normal woman." It took Letitia another ten years to recognize that her husband was the one who had the problem, and she finally found the courage to leave this man. However, Letitia still carries doubts about her ability to "be a woman to a man." She told me that she had no intentions of ever having another partner relationship, because she was "frightened that it would destroy my image of myself as a complete woman."

Regardless of whether respondents were heterosexual, lesbian, or bisexual, the quality of their relationships with intimate partners was the most significant factor in their stated ability to maintain or reclaim gender identity following surgery. Supportive partners, both female and male, not only provided much needed material help, but their emotional support was also crucial to affirming that respondents were still women, despite missing organs. Conversely, rejecting partners, all male, were detrimental to women's confidence in their ability to maintain or reclaim their gender identity following gynecological surgery. These conclusions again emphasize the interaction between biological and social factors in the preservation of gender identity.

8

"Am I Still a Woman?"

We all need help in learning the obvious . . . that women are made, not born; women are born, not made; and that both statements are true in their profound and limited fashion.

—*Natalie Angier,* Woman: An Intimate Geography

The body can never be regarded merely as a site of quantifiable processes that can be assessed objectively, but must be treated as invested with personal meaning, history, and value that are ultimately determinable only by the subject who lives 'within' it.

—*Susan Bordo,* Unbearable Weight

THIS BOOK has explored the experiences of forty-four American women who have undergone hysterectomy, with or without oophorectomy, for benign conditions. Hysterectomy is a crisis that offers a unique opportunity to contemplate the meaning of sexual/reproductive organs in the context of female identity. It is tempting to demand that the data produce a definitive answer to a specific question: *Does gynecological surgery produce a change in gender identity?* Nevertheless, I have made it clear from the beginning that I did not approach this research with the expectation that respondents who had widely differing social backgrounds and experiences would react in similar ways simply because they underwent the same medical procedures. My findings confirm that some women believe that their bodies and lives have been greatly altered by surgery, others sense very little change, and some perceive no change at all. The one consistent factor for all forty-four respondents was that gynecological surgery was a reason for reflection about gender identity.

So, Do Respondents Feel They Are Still Women?

Yes, No, Maybe

As I discussed at length in Chapter 1, the term *woman* can be used to represent biology, socialization, role performance, or discourse. Since respondents used the term in each of these ways, I have reflected the multiple meanings of *woman* in my discussion. For most respondents, the answer to the question "Am I still a woman?" was not as simple as "yes" or "no." These women had more nuanced understandings of the effect of gynecological surgery on their own gender identities.

In some cases, this effect was determined by the material fact of whether respondents had simple hysterectomies or their surgeries also included the removal of their ovaries (as I discussed in Chapters 2 and 3). For other respondents, abstract factors were more important, including the subjective meanings they associated with menstruation (Chapter 4), childbearing (Chapter 5), and sexuality (Chapter 6). While most respondents did not feel diminished as women because they no longer menstruated, the preponderance of those who were premenopausal at the time of surgery believed that loss of fertility did impair their gender identity. Respondents' perceptions of the impact of hysterectomy and oophorectomy on their sexuality were more diverse than their reactions to the end of menstruation or fertility. This includes women who believe that their identities either as sexual objects or sexual subjects remained unchanged, those for whom sexual relations were worse following surgery, and those for whom it was better.

Factors Influencing Disruption of Gender Identity

Throughout this book, I have analyzed the symbolic gender meanings that women may associate with their uteruses and ovaries.

Although the significance of losing sexual reproductive organs varied among respondents, some general themes are prevalent. On the whole, those respondents who were more likely to suffer disrupted gender identities were:

1. *Women who underwent bilateral salpingo-oophorectomy (bs-o) as well as hysterectomy.* Because the ovaries are closely associated with the production of "female" hormones, bs-o often carried greater symbolic meanings for respondents' gender identities than did hysterectomy alone. Respondents whose ovaries were removed were therefore more likely to question their gender normalcy following surgery. This was particularly true if they had been premenopausal prior to bs-o and surgery had initiated an untimely and abrupt surgical menopause (see Chapters 2 and 3).

2. *Women who were considered still fertile prior to surgery, regardless of whether they had already given birth.* A significant consequence of hysterectomy is that it renders a previously (at least hypothetically) fertile woman infertile. Not all respondents regretted the loss of their reproductive capability. A small number, for various reasons, were actually relieved that after hysterectomy they would never again need to worry about becoming pregnant. However, the preponderance of respondents were distressed by becoming infertile. While childless women were most upset by this, premenopausal women with children were also strongly affected by the permanent and premature closing of their potential for further childbearing, not only before they were psychologically ready but also before they were sociologically ready in relationship to their age cohort. Furthermore, some women who previously had no desire to give birth were dismayed that they were no longer in control of their own childbearing decisions. It is the *potential* ability to gestate a child that is terminated with the removal of the uterus, and it is that loss of potential that is mourned as an impairment to gender identity (see Chapter 5).

3. *Heterosexual women who feared diminished sexual attractiveness and who did not have supportive partners, as well as women, regardless of sexual preference, who perceived negative changes in sexual response.*

Sexuality is a basic component of gender identity. This involves the ability to act both as an appropriate sexual object and as a capable sexual subject. Respondents who expressed fears regarding possible diminished sexual attractiveness were predominantly heterosexual. Cultural standards that they perceived were problematic after surgery included a youthful appearance, a slim figure, and physical flawlessness. In addition, several women believed that just the fact of having undergone hysterectomy was a discreditable stigma that had the potential to spoil their gender identities as appropriate sexual objects. Supportive partners helped to mitigate these fears, whereas rejecting partners reinforced doubts. Several respondents—heterosexual, lesbian, and bisexual—noted negative changes in either libido or sexual pleasure following gynecological surgery, which detracted from their perceived ability to be "complete women." (See Chapter 6.)

4. *Women who believed that they had no control over decisions to undergo surgery.* Respondents were less able to deal with perceived threats to their gender identity after surgery if they believed that they had not been offered alternatives and did not have the prior opportunity to consider the subjective meanings of gynecological surgery (discussed further in this chapter).

These generalizations cannot be regarded as universal, even for my sample. I found contrary examples of women who felt great losses to their gender identity despite being past menopause, retaining both ovaries, having supportive partners, and believing that it was their own choice to have hysterectomies. Correspondingly, some women perceived no gender losses even though they were premenopausal, lost both ovaries, and did not have supportive partners. However, these were exceptions.

Alternative Identity Possibilities

When I began this project, I considered the possibility that, since the uterus and ovaries are so strongly connected to women's gender identity, respondents might describe bodily changes that resulted from gynecological surgery as opportunities for transformations into alternative sex and gender identities. Cross-cultural comparisons present possibilities for more than two constructed categories of gender (Kessler and McKenna 1978). I speculated that respondents might envision themselves as "neuters," "liminal figures," or members of a "third sex." In fact, some women did place themselves within these categories, but this group represents a distinct minority.

Neuter

If sexual organs define *woman*, as biological essentialist discourse claims, an individual who does not have a uterus and/or ovaries cannot qualify as one. However, she cannot qualify as *man*, either, because she does not possess the requisite organs for that identity. Some medical authorities have suggested that even a naturally menopausal woman with intact organs is "not really a man but no longer a woman" (Wilson and Wilson 1963, qtd. in Fausto-Sterling 1985, 110–11). If this presumption is considered, respondents might certainly wonder about their own postsurgery gender status. Terry told me that, although she had never felt that her sexual/reproductive organs were an important part of her identity, "the absence thereof really was devastating. I really felt castrated. I really felt neutered in many ways." Although for Terry this was simply an initial perception, Isabella continued to feel this way at the time of our interview. Although she did not consider herself a man, she referred to herself as no longer a woman, simply a "fake woman."

Liminal Figure

Anthropologist Victor Turner defines *liminality* as "'betwixt and between the positions assigned and arrayed by law, custom, convention and ceremonial'" (1969, 45). Individuals reach this state by moving from "an earlier fixed point in the social structure" (44), and thus they "embody disorder" (Smith-Rosenberg 1985, 151). Performance theory describes *liminality* as a "virtual space" in which transformation and play can take place. Actors move in and out of the liminal space, which is always available for agents to enter and exit (Turnbull 1985). Conceivably, the "disordered" bodies of women who do not have uteruses or ovaries might be perceived as *liminal.*

Frances regarded "no longer being totally a woman" as an asset. She told me that she felt she did not have to identify with either a male or female identity: "So it's kind of like . . . you kind of pick the pieces of different genders that you want to have or different behaviors. . . . I think the only person who puts boundaries on us is us." Frances therefore believed that her post-hysterectomy body allowed her to take greater advantage of identifying with both male and female identities. She could perform either or both when she wanted to. For example, this was the way Frances interpreted having the ability to engage in sexual intercourse without the risk of getting pregnant. Some theorists (i.e., Foucault 1980) propose that hermaphrodites occupy liminal space, possessing some male and some female physical characteristics. It would be interesting to imagine hermaphrodites and hysterectomized individuals sharing liminal space, since one is seen as having a surplus of sexual reproductive organs, the other as having a deficit.[1]

Third Sex

Fausto-Sterling (1993) maintains that two sexes are not enough to describe the variety of human sexual identities. Perhaps, then, women without sexual reproductive organs might see themselves as neither male nor female but as members of a third category. Other marginalized subjects have previously appropriated this third category. For example, Carl Ulrichs, who argued for nineteenth-century homosexual rights, described gay men as "'a third sex' in whom the soul of a woman was trapped in the body of a man" (Meyer 1991, 33). So maybe hysterectomized women might identify with a fourth or fifth category of gender. This additional category might be an androgynous one, combining both male and female components, or it might be a completely different identity. However, none of the women I interviewed perceived themselves as members of an additional sex or gender category. Instead, their narratives endorsed the cultural binary divisions of sex and gender.

Gender Rebels and Conservators

Despite the few exceptions noted above, it is notable that the overwhelming majority of respondents still consider themselves *women*. The results of this study strongly indicate that cultural gender identity norms are enduring. As documented by Kessler and McKenna, in current American culture "'I don't know' or 'Neither' or 'Both' are not acceptable answers" to the question of personal gender identity—in order to be regarded as human, an individual must be assigned to one of the two binary sex and gender categories (1978, 8). Notwithstanding their descriptions of specific losses to gender identity, nearly all respondents asserted that they still identify as women. Although postmodern theorists might object to the idea of surrendering identity to a constructed category of gender, the individuals that I interviewed, like most contemporary women, are not postmodern.[2] They placed great value on their ability to identify as women.

Nevertheless, in claiming female and feminine identities, respondents are not simply passive recipients of cultural prescriptions; they exercise agency by stretching biological definitions of *womanhood*. These individuals claimed that they were women both because they once retained female sexual reproductive organs and also in spite of their current lack of them. In so doing, respondents acted both as gender conservators and as gender rebels. This might confirm Connell's theory (1987) that "denials," "transformations," and "contradictions" can open the categories of gender. However, the forms of evidence that respondents employed to argue that they are still women merely demonstrate the extent to which gender and sex, culture and biology, are still very much intertwined.

Cultural Essentialist Arguments

Almost all respondents adopted aspects of the "natural attitude" regarding gender identity (Garfinkel 1967, 122–28; Howard and Hollander 1997, 35–36; Kessler and McKenna 1978, 113–14). This includes cultural assumptions that there are two and only two genders but also that gender identity never varies once it is established. Respondents repeatedly told me that they *had* to be women because they knew they weren't men, and having always thought of themselves as female, it was inconceivable that they could be anything else. As Kessler and McKenna note, in our dualistic construction of sex and gender, the identities *male* and *female* are "mutually constitutive," and almost nothing can discredit a gender attribution once it is made (1978, 159). These theorists affirm that "even the loss of the original criteria [in this case, uteruses and ovaries] used to make the attribution might well become irrelevant" (160). In addition to claiming female identity because they had once possessed uteruses and ovaries, a few respondents rested their claims on the fact that they still had breasts and vaginas. Interestingly, no respondent referred to her female chromosomes as evidence that she is a woman.

The few respondents who believe that they no longer qualify as women adhere to a strict biological essentialist understanding of sex and gender. An example of this was Bernadette, who told me, "I feel like I'm not a whole woman anymore . . . just that, and you're missing something, you're lacking something that a woman should have." While *biological* essentialist arguments such as that one might be problematic for respondents who do believe that they are still women, the respondents generally uphold *cultural* essentialist arguments to prove their case. As I discuss in Chapter 1, biological essentialist theories define *women* by their biological or "natural" characteristics. However, cultural essentialist arguments connect women's essence to personality characteristics that are presumed to be universal, including "nurturance, empathy, supportiveness, noncompetitiveness," or certain ways of acting, including "intuitiveness, emotional responses, concern and commitment to helping others" (Grosz 1994, 84). The essentialist assumption is that males and females evidence strictly defined and identifiable characteristics that can be created by nature or by nurture.

A significant number of respondents base their claim that they are women on what they consider fundamental female personality traits. For example, Ernestine told me:

A woman is a being who is blessed with sensitivity and doesn't have to be ashamed to be sensitive, as opposed to men. . . . A woman, whether she has children or not, is often a mother, a guider, and a listener. These mother traits go into your other relationships, too.

Indeed, even Susan, who had a professional career and had never been a mother, professed:

> For me, my womanliness is bound up in how I view loving kindness. I identify that more with women than I do with men. . . . For me, it's playing the conscience of the family, the social role and also the source of loving and considerate behavior toward my extended family. I don't think of myself as the breadwinner, or the fixer, or the person everybody turns to in times of trouble for sage advice. I'm more the person who keeps things together, keeps people in connection with one another . . . the heart and soul of the family. . . . I see it that way . . . I do what I can do, to try to play that role as closely as I can, even though I can't play it out the way a mother does.

Caring for others, being sensitive, and not being afraid to show strong emotions were frequently mentioned as evidence by respondents that they were "still women."

In Chapter 7 I discussed respondents' use of impression management to clearly indicate their gender identity to others as well as to reinforce it for themselves. Women actively created their preferred gender identities through selecting certain behaviors and appearances. Thus, although Howard and Hollander (1997) assert that principles of symbolic interaction are incompatible with essentialist approaches to gender, they presumably refer only to *biological* essentialism. I found that impression management was an effective strategy to contextualize respondents' reinscription of *cultural* essence.

While respondents paid great attention to performing female identities, a crucial piece of evidence supporting their claims to womanhood is the fact that they once did have uteruses and ovaries. As I explained in Chapter 1, Judith Butler's concept of performance theory (1990) is an extreme view of the enactment of gender. She asserts that all gender is merely performance and theorizes that gender can completely escape the concept of a material body. To the contrary, respondents in my study ground their claims to female identity in (former) biological fact. Actually, it could be argued that someone who has had a hysterectomy *must* be a woman, because only women can undergo this surgery.[3] As I listened to respondents' descriptions of their surgical experiences, I began to realize that gynecological surgery can be conceptualized as a particular form of "doing gender." Respondents identified with several cultural constructions of gender, including those that view female bodies as unstable and defective, as objectified, and as powerless.

Gynecological Surgery as a Form of "Doing Gender"

Constructions of Female Bodies as Unstable and Defective

The first way in which respondents discussed gynecological surgery as a form of "doing gender" was by implying that their hysterectomies had been necessary because their bodies, like other female bodies, were inherently unstable and defective. Historically, medical discourse has played a crucial role in this social construction of female identity (Bush 1999; Ussher 1992), and contemporary medical discourse continues to describe female bodies as unstable and fundamentally uncontrollable unless closely monitored (Lupton 1994). This message is reinforced and disseminated to women through the popular media as women are constantly warned about the potential diseases inherent in their internal sexual reproductive organs. It is hardly surprising, then, that many respondents saw hysterectomy as an inevitable part of being a woman. Several women, especially the older ones, told me that they knew so many other women who had hysterectomies that they felt it was almost routine. So many of May's friends had undergone gynecological surgery at about the same time she did (in approximately 1938), that she joked, "Hysterectomies are contagious, you know."

In the context of cultural understandings, most respondents were haunted by the specter of female bodies that would inevitably go further and further out of control, either hemorrhaging, causing unbearable pain, or, most frightening of all, developing cancer. Yvonne told me that that she was distressed when she found out that she had fibroid tumors (a common benign condition) because she remembered her neighbor being rushed to the hospital to have an emergency hysterectomy due to hemorrhaging caused by fibroids. Yvonne commented that, after an office visit where her gynecologist told her that her fibroids had gotten bigger:

> I think, as I recall, the only thing he said was that they [the fibroid tumors] could only get worse. And when he said "worse," I think I extrapolated the hemorrhaging. I think that's what I knew from this neighbor, and I knew that I had [fibroids] for a while and that I had been sent to a surgeon [previously] and more or less escaped. And I think probably I decided that this was the end of the line, and I had postponed it [hysterectomy] and now I'm at this point that it needs to be done. . . . As I said, I think this neighbor really played a strong influence on it. And I knew that my father's sister had had to have one [hysterectomy] because of fibroids, and I think that she had hemorrhaging problems too. So I think I just put that whole mix together and thought, *"I guess it's time, it's inevitable."*

A number of respondents told me that what led to their hysterectomies was "woman problems," a generic term that was employed as a euphemism for gynecological difficulties. I was prompted to wonder whether "woman problems" not only implied problems that women may have but also that respondents perceived that *being* a woman in and of itself may be a problem.

Several respondents had close family members or friends who had undergone hysterectomies and thus were not surprised when it was "their time." During our interview, Penny conferred with her sister (who was in the room) about the members of their family who had undergone hysterectomies: "Oh yeah, you had one, Auntie Peg had one, Sally had one, and three of her sisters had them." Similarly, Brooke commented that her mother told her, "Oh, well, you're just like all the other Miller women . . . and three-quarters of them had—I mean, it was rare if someone *didn't* have a hysterectomy!" Wendy informed me that she "learned that there are a lot of 'woman problems' that run in my family. My sister had all kinds of problems. Bleeding, bleeding for days. That runs in the women in the family. So, again, I just thought it was part of what I inherited."

Joy was not surprised when her daughter developed a number of gynecological problems because, as she explained, "I feel the apple doesn't fall far from the tree." Joy told me that she is glad that her granddaughter is adopted because she believes that her lack of genetic connection means that she might not experience similar gynecological difficulties. These women discussed the problems leading to their hysterectomies as a sort of female family curse that is passed from mother to daughter.

Hysterectomy is usually considered the final solution to many gynecological dilemmas. If female bodies are at risk of going out of control, gynecologists are given the authority to monitor those bodies and to take action to restrain them. Gynecologists appear to consider it their mission to rescue women from dangerous uteruses and ovaries. For example, Dr. Christiane Northrup (1998) reveals that her medical training included socialization into what she refers to as "our cultural inheritance." This included being told aphorisms such as, "There's no room in the tomb for the womb" and "The uterus is for growing babies or for growing cancer." She also reports that hysterectomies were commonly performed only for "chronic and persistent uterus" (Northrup 1998, 166). This rhetoric frames physicians' perceptions of women's sexual reproductive organs—perceptions that they pass along to their female patients. Most respondents did not question their gynecologists' decisions that they needed hysterectomies. This was particularly true for women who had surgery more than twenty years ago, including May, who told me: "When there's things wrong with your female organs, then the doctors have to do what's right."

Some respondents suspected that the real reason they received hysterectomies was because, as women, unrelated physical problems were attributed to their sexual reproductive organs. Allison's experience is a case in point. She is now convinced that the hemorrhaging that prompted her emergency hysterectomy and bs-o at age 28 was not a gynecological problem at all, but a bleeding disorder that was later diagnosed by a hematologist. She told me that she believes that physicians follow scripts when they see uncontrolled bleeding in women, and that they simply assume that any internal problems that women have are gynecological in nature.

Sarah is also dubious regarding the rationale for her surgery. Almost immediately after undergoing the hysterectomy that was supposed to be the solution to the unremitting pain she had experienced for several years, her pain returned. She told me:

> Come to find out, it was the gall bladder that was causing the severe pain. I was having gall bladder attacks! And they never looked at that. They were looking much lower, at my lower organs, and they never thought of the gall bladder. Never!! I cannot believe that!

Although her symptoms had not included heavy bleeding or other menstrual problems, Sarah perceived that the doctors she consulted with were "targeting" her uterus. She now believes that doctors might have paid more attention to her symptoms if she had been a man: "I don't think a man ever would have been treated like that, ever. . . . I think it has to do with the fact that women aren't valued as high. And I think I felt a little of that in my own upbringing, that somehow I wasn't as important."

The cultural concept that women's bodies are inherently unstable and defective may influence physicians to assume that the origin of a multitude of physical problems is gynecological. This assumption induces them to perform hysterectomies for problems whose causation lies elsewhere.

Constructions of Female Bodies as Objects

A second way in which respondents referred to hysterectomy as a form of "doing gender" was their view that they had been treated, like other women, as objects. Previous research (Fisher 1986; Scully 1994; Todd 1989) confirms that, due to women's generally lower social status, many gynecologists fail to treat them as autonomous subjects. Moreover, since women commonly experience cultural objectification of their bodies, they may be vulnerable to expecting this treatment by physicians. Some respondents have learned to be more assertive about medical care since their surgeries, like Yvonne, who told me that she would definitely ask more questions now than she had at the time of her hysterectomy in 1973 and her bs-o in 1986. However, most respondents, even those who underwent surgery very recently, did not feel entitled to engage in a dialogue with their doctors.

Ernestine expressed the sentiments of a number of respondents when she asserted that her surgeon treated her "like an object." This is apparently a common perspective among gynecological patients. Emily Martin discusses the "separation of self from body that women describe when they talk about menstruation, menopause, and birth" and that is "present to an extreme degree when they describe cesarean section" (1992, 79). I found that an even more extreme degree of objectification might occur for women who believe that their own body parts are attacking them and that they need gynecological surgery to save themselves from their defective and aggressive uteruses and ovaries. Martin asserts that "somehow being referred to as a 'section' after a cesarean does not help a woman feel like a whole person" (82). Analogously, several women in my study reported the alienation they felt when they overheard hospital staff referring to them as a "hyst" following their hysterectomies.

When the individual views her own body, not as part of her integrated person, but as an object, she is more likely to rely on professional expertise to fix it. For example, Ann compared feeling better after her hysterectomy and bs-o to repairing her car: "You know, like when your car breaks down and if you have an old car, you don't quite realize what a piece of shit it is until you drive a new car."

In a few cases, women were *literally* objects rather than sentient beings, since their doctors made surgical decisions regarding hysterectomy unilaterally while they were under general anesthesia.

Although all but one of these women had signed general consent forms when admitted for exploratory surgery, they later expressed surprise that their doctors had actually removed their uteruses and ovaries for anything besides cancer. Deborah, who did sign a general consent form but was told that it was highly unlikely that she would undergo hysterectomy and oophorectomy, was angry with her physician afterwards because "he made this decision just to take my 'woman-ness' away from me during surgery." Janet's surgeon performed a total hysterectomy and bs-o during exploratory laparoscopy,[4] despite the fact that she had never consented to these procedures. The medical excuse for expanded surgery in each of these cases was that the doctor had seen more extensive damage than was expected and was therefore saving the patient from hypothetical future surgery. However, all of these women believed that they should have been revived from anesthesia and consulted before undergoing such drastic surgery for benign conditions. Like the women in Martin's study who underwent cesarean sections when they had expected vaginal births, these respondents had strong feelings of being "forcibly violated" while helpless to defend themselves.[5]

Some respondents who complained about being dehumanized by their surgeons speculated that the gender of their physicians might have influenced the extent of their surgeries. They reasoned that male gynecologists might have a cavalier attitude about removing uteruses and ovaries because they themselves don't have these body parts. Letitia commented on the poor medical treatment she received: "I think it's a male thing, a male doctor thing, or just a male thing." Gloria believed that having a feminist woman doctor made an important difference in preserving an ovary during hysterectomy. And Charlotte told me that since her hysterectomy she would only go to a woman doctor because "female doctors know what you're going through—sometimes male doctors are 'Oh, yeah, OK' . . . but they really don't understand."

It seems logical that female physicians might be less likely to interpret hysterectomy and oophorectomy as simply the removal of extraneous body parts and also might be more likely to see their female patients as whole individuals. However, several respondents gave examples demonstrating that shared gender does not necessarily make female physicians more empathetic. Barbara blames her emergency hysterectomy on the fact that her female gynecologist refused to see her during the preceding weeks, despite her severe bleeding problems. Likewise, when Sarah was in tremendous pain following hysterectomy, her female physician callously told her, "I guess you're going to have to learn to tolerate the pain." Sarah complained that she could not get this doctor to see her in the weeks following surgery and that at her six-week checkup, when she was still suffering, "she dropped me like I was a hot potato. She didn't want to see me any more." As previous research has found, medical socialization can be stronger than gender socialization (Fugh-Berman 1994; Lorber 2000). Apparently, female physicians may be just as susceptible to negative cultural constructions of women's bodies as are their male colleagues and equally insensitive to the subjectivity of their patients.

Constructions of Female Bodies as Powerless

A third way in which respondents perceived hysterectomy as a form of "doing gender" was based on their feelings of powerlessness regarding possible options. Feminists have long argued in favor of women's rights to control their own bodies. Choice is a crucial element not only in the examples of birth control and abortion but in the case of gynecological surgery as well. Many women I interviewed told me that the decision to undergo hysterectomy was their "own choice." However, this decision was filtered through their physicians' advice regarding currently available medical options. For example, Letitia told me that at the time she decided to undergo gynecological surgery, she had "no idea" what a hysterectomy was, "except that I knew there was relief someplace."

For many respondents, various other surgical and drug treatments for pain and bleeding had already failed to help. These women believed that they had simply run out of options, and it was not a matter of *if* they would need a hysterectomy—it was only a matter of *when* they would have it. As Terry put it, "My body made the decision for me." Although hysterectomy was not something she would have chosen if she could have avoided it, she thought about it for a long time and felt that "it came to me out of a real physical necessity. It was something I had to attend to if I wanted to have a decent quality of life." Christine complained that, although she had in fact read a lot of feminist critiques regarding hysterectomy as an "unnecessary operation done on women so that men can put women down," at the time of her surgery she had the more immediate concern of stopping her vaginal hemorrhaging and was offered no alternatives.

Several women told me that they had been bleeding heavily and almost constantly before surgery or that they were in so much pain that they could barely function and just wanted to be "normal" again. To these women, life without a uterus and/or ovaries seemed more "normal" than life with unbearable bleeding and/or pain. For example, Arlene said: "I was just so happy I'd had the operation." And Page told me that after her hysterectomy, "I felt so terrific. I couldn't believe how wonderful I felt—fabulous—I didn't realize how bad I had been feeling." Madison explained that she "had no regrets. It was a big relief." She wished she'd had a hysterectomy sooner "instead of futzing around for a couple of years." Some of these women lionized their gynecological surgeons as heroes who had saved them from the future misery their problematic female parts might have caused. Frances, Sunny, and Kelly all used the words "love" and "trust" when referring to the feelings they had towards their surgeons.

Some women were particularly adamant that they had been active agents who made fully informed choices regarding hysterectomy. They resented any implication that there were drawbacks to surgery. For example, Ann told me that she "got a lot of really obnoxious unsolicited advice from people who were really ideologically opposed to [hysterectomy]." She was angry with women who implied that she had been "bamboozled by the medical establishment" into having a hysterectomy when all she felt was relief. Similarly, Frances maintained that if women have gynecological problems, even at a young age, they should not hesitate to undergo hysterectomy. She believed these women should not be told, "You're going to end up losing the essence of what it means to be a woman"; they should just "get on with it."

Other respondents concluded that, even though they had previously thought surgery had been their own personal choice, they had not really understood what the implications would be, nor had they been given the opportunity to consider how they might feel emotionally afterwards. Isabella told me that if she had it to do over again, despite her bleeding and pain, she would tell the surgeon, "No, I don't want to take it [her uterus] out, leave it like that." Alice, who had expected to feel relief after hysterectomy, found that there were downsides she hadn't anticipated, but "it was done, it was over, and now I had to live with it."

Joy (whose hysterectomy was in 1968) explained, "At that stage I still had the attitude that doctors knew it all." Ethel (who underwent hysterectomy and bs-o in 1969) told me that, when she tried to discuss options to hysterectomy with her "arrogant" surgeon, he remarked, "I got my education from Princeton and Johns Hopkins, did you get yours from *Reader's Digest*?" Although she "felt like smacking him," Ethel politely went along with the surgery he recommended because, she said, "I think I was raised in a time when women weren't thought of as being as intelligent as men and that we should accept male authority."

In addition to the normal consequences of hysterectomy, a fairly large number of women I interviewed developed iatrogenic problems resulting from surgery. These included high fever, breathing problems, staph infections, anemia, painful adhesions, urinary infections, bladder prolapse, internal hemorrhaging, pneumonia, abscess, infection, gangrene, peritonitis, burst appendix, cardiac arrest, collapsed lung, intestinal damage, perforated bowel, hepatitis, blood clots in legs, and extreme weight loss. These surgical outcomes led women to reexamine their previous decisions to undergo hysterectomy, perceiving that the cure may have been worse than their previous symptoms. After terrible surgical complications that almost killed her and that required eight additional surgeries and almost a year in the hospital, Letitia complained, "They don't take women seriously . . . so . . . why bother to try to find another treatment for it?"

Although most hysterectomies are considered "elective" procedures, it is important to ask whether they are "elective from the viewpoint of the patient or that of the physician" (Travis 1985, 250). At least two respondents were particularly suspicious about whether they had been persuaded to agree to have hysterectomies for which there was no real physical justification. One of these was Lupe, whose gynecologist had informed her that she had to undergo hysterectomy because her uterus was dangerously enlarged, even though she felt no symptoms. When this physician visited her in the hospital after her surgery, Lupe asked him what had been wrong with her uterus, and he replied that it was still being analyzed at the lab. Although her hysterectomy was two and a half years before our interview, Lupe's doctor had never been able to find her medical reports at any postoperative visits. A friend who worked in the lab told her he "checked out" the report on her uterus and said, "Nothing was wrong with it . . . everything was normal. There was nothing wrong inside. You had no tumors. No nothing. There was nothing wrong with it." This prompted Lupe to belatedly reassess her decision to undergo hysterectomy, which had been based on her physician's advice that she needed one:

> I'm thinking "Was this really necessary now?" Could it have been taken care of through medication? So I'm still in the mind of thinking "OK, I was part of another screw-up . . ." So I said, "Fine. I just don't want to see this doctor's face any more," because I swear I think I would have strangled him.

Lupe regretted that she didn't just get up and walk away from the hospital, as she considered doing before she was "knocked out" with anesthesia. However, she also felt helpless to do anything about it after the fact.

Anita also became skeptical about the necessity for her hysterectomy. At her six-week postpartum checkup after the birth of twins (her fourth and fifth children at the age of 27), her gynecologist told Anita that she had to have a hysterectomy or she "would die." Since her mother had died young, Anita readily agreed to the surgery, which was scheduled immediately. Anita told me that, after her hysterectomy, "I started thinking, and I said to myself, 'Could this be possible that he could be a bad doctor, trying to get money [from Medicaid] or something?'" Her suspicions heightened when about a month later she read in the newspaper that her surgeon was arrested for doing unnecessary "welfare surgeries." Then, Anita told me, "I freaked. I said, 'Maybe I didn't even have to have this!'"

Whether women saw themselves as passive victims or as active agents, free choice to undergo a hysterectomy can only be constrained choice, at best. Even respondents who claimed that they had welcomed hysterectomy and were completely satisfied with the results were constrained by a lack of alternative options. They often explained that desperation had driven them to undergo hysterectomy in order to alleviate their gynecological problems but that they would have preferred less radical options if those had been offered. Most of the women I interviewed would probably agree with Deborah, who commented: "I wish there were ways of dealing with [gynecological problems] that didn't distort your body so much." The power to choose is meaningless if women are given no alternatives. Thus, respondents' feelings of powerlessness regarding choices made about their bodies, experiences of being objectified by physicians, and perceptions of their female bodies as unstable and defective combine to construct hysterectomy as an explicit form of "doing" female gender.

Implications for a Combined Perspective of Gender Identity

An important research goal in undertaking this study was to further elucidate the complicated interactions between the material body and the social body as elaborated by respondents' perceptions regarding their lived experiences of gynecological surgery. In Chapter 1, I explained that most theories regarding gender identity begin with the assumption that either "anatomy is destiny" or social factors render biology moot. Feminist sociology has faced a dilemma in reconciling material bodies with the concept that bodies are socially constructed. James Weinrich (1990) provides a possible resolution. He asserts that both biological and social perspectives can be simultaneously correct. While it is obvious that extreme forms of each position are mutually incompatible, Weinrich maintains that more moderate social constructionist and biological theories "interact in a way that is more than the sum of their parts" (182). Using the analogy of how the degree of skin tanning depends on the interaction between the biological factor of skin color and the social factor of sun exposure, he demonstrates that biology and social practice are jointly determined.[6]

Elizabeth Grosz (1994) suggests applying the möbius strip analogy to theories about the human body. A möbius strip is a twisted three-dimensional figure eight on which the outside and the inside become continuous, constantly merging. The inside surface of the möbius strip can represent the biological and phenomenological aspects of the body, while the outside can correspond to social and cultural aspects. The möbius strip is thus a model for transcending dualistic conceptions regarding bodily experience.

My study lends support for a combined approach to theorizing gender identity. I discovered that, disconnected from each other, strictly biological, cultural, or social constructionist theories provide inadequate explanations of women's hysterectomy experiences. Respondents continually merged biological, cultural, and social rationales to assert that they are still *women* or (in a few cases) to deny that they are still *women*. The interweaving of biological, social, and cultural understandings in their narratives demonstrates the "both/and" (rather than "either/or") character of embodied gender identity. A combined biological, cultural, and social constructionist perspective could also provide enhanced insight into the connection between masculine gender identity and surgery that affects men's sexual reproductive organs (e.g., prostatectomy and orchiectomy).

Postscript

The Issue of Medical Necessity

IT IS NEARLY impossible to discuss gynecological surgery without mentioning the issue of unnecessary surgery. Indeed, this aspect has been the primary emphasis in previous feminist research on hysterectomy. The fact that many hysterectomies and oophorectomies are performed for inappropriate reasons is implicit in my discussion of respondents' narratives, although that is not the main emphasis of this book.

For at least the past fifty years, women's health advocates have leveled the charge that many hysterectomies are unnecessary. More recently, the responsible medical community has also admitted that the American hysterectomy rate is excessive. Previously, the putative motivation for unnecessary surgery was that it was an artifact of fee-for-service medical plans whereby physicians were financially rewarded for performing expensive surgery. However, cost-cutting measures by managed care organizations have not appreciably decreased hysterectomies.

RAND, an independent, nonprofit research organization, conducted a study of gynecological surgery for the Agency for Health Care Policy and Research of the U.S. Department of Health and Human Services (Bernstein et al. 1997). This study used a panel of nine medical experts in gynecology to establish an "appropriateness" scale for hysterectomy, rating reasons for hysterectomy as "appropriate," "uncertain," and "inappropriate." The scale was used to rate hysterectomies performed on 642 randomly selected women who had undergone hysterectomies through seven health maintenance organizations nationwide. According to the medical panel, only 58 percent of the hysterectomies studied had been performed for appropriate reasons. Moreover, among women under forty years of age, only 44 percent of hysterectomies were rated "appropriate" (Brody 1993). In addition, a February 2000 article in *Obstetrics and Gynecology* reported that 70 percent of hysterectomies performed on women enrolled in Southern California managed care organizations (MCOs) between 1993 and 1995 were done for reasons that did not meet American College of Obstetricians and Gynecologists (ACOG) criteria. The most prevalent reasons that these hysterectomies were considered unnecessary were lack of sufficient diagnostic evaluation and failure to attempt alternative treatments (National Women's Health Network 2001).

Decisions regarding gynecological surgery are not based completely on objective data. In fact, the probability that a woman will undergo hysterectomy may depend more on sociological than on medical reasons. Social characteristics—including age, social class, race, educational attainment, welfare status, number of abortions, unwed motherhood, and type of medical coverage—are often determining factors as to who will undergo hysterectomy (Fisher 1986; Kjerulff, Langenberg and Guzinkis 1993; Meilahn et al. 1989).[1]

As mentioned in Chapter 1, the American hysterectomy rate is three to four times higher than in Australia, New Zealand, and almost all European countries (Lepine 1997). In addition, rates vary widely within the United States; the hysterectomy rate is almost twice as high in the South as in the Northeast despite lack of evidence that uterine disease is more common in one region than in another (Franklin 1991). Rates vary more locally as well. In the northeastern state where most respondents in my study live, the hysterectomy rate was as much as five times greater in some small geographic areas than in others between 1982 and 1989 (Bernstein et al. 1997). Differences in hysterectomy rates may arise from "differences in physician training, the style of medical practice in an area, or even availability of gynecologists and hospital beds," according to Franklin (1991, 603). An article in the *New England Journal of Medicine* (Carlson, Nichols, Schiff 1993) acknowledges that "variations in hysterectomy rates are caused by a wide variety of factors including patient characteristics, availability of medical resources and professional attitudes." However, the possible individual subjective significance of sexual reproductive organs is not generally explored prior to surgery.

Hysterectomy and oophorectomy are permanent. Currently, there are no replacements for uteruses and ovaries, although medical researchers have made attempts to create them. Early-twentieth-century physicians first tried to transplant ovaries in order to relieve menopausal symptoms, but they discontinued these experiments when synthesized hormone replacement therapies were developed (Squier 2000). In 1999 medical researchers announced that they had begun to successfully reimplant pieces of previously removed and frozen ovaries (Weiss 1999), but there is doubt as to whether these transplants will actually function long-term.

Scientists have made attempts at transplanting uteruses in animals since the 1950s, but they have ultimately been unsuccessful. In the March 7, 2002 issue of the *International Journal of Gynecology and Obstetrics,* surgeons from Saudi Arabia announced that they had performed the first human uterine transplant in April 2000 (Fageeh, Raffa, Jabbad, and Mazouki 2002). A donor organ from a 46-year-old Yemenite woman (who had previously undergone bs-o for ovarian cysts) was transplanted into a 26-year-old Saudi woman whose uterus had been removed six years earlier due to uncontrolled bleeding following the birth of her first child.[2] The uterine transplantation was extremely difficult because many tiny blood vessels had to be reattached with microsurgical techniques, and the uterus recipient was required to take immune system suppressing drugs to avoid organ rejection. The transplanted uterus produced two menstrual periods until it was removed after ninety-nine days due to complications involving blood clots, just when surgeons were preparing to attempt in vitro fertilization. Despite this, the surgeons reported that the transplant was essentially successful. An editorial in the same medical journal concluded that this case should not be regarded as a failure; reproductive organs are the "new frontier" in transplant surgery. The editorial further speculated that in the near future women who have undergone hysterectomy will be able to become pregnant and gestate their own babies with transplanted uteruses (Grady 2002b). However, other medical specialists, in both the transplant and fertility fields, firmly contend that costs and ethical issues make it unlikely that uterine transplantation will ever become a viable alternative in the United States (Smith 2002).

Also in the winter of 2002, a scientist at Cornell University announced that he had enabled a human embryo to develop on the wall of artificially engineered tissue simulating the inside of a uterus.[3] This experiment was halted after six days, and the supervising scientist cautions that researchers are far from simulating an entire external artificial womb (Cook 2002).

There are many ethical issues regarding the question of whether medical science should continue to work toward the goal of transplanting ovaries, transplanting uteruses, or creating artificial wombs. These "cures" might make hysterectomy and oophorectomy even more commonplace if sexual reproductive organs would then be regarded as replaceable. This potential situation might not actually meet women's subjective needs. However, if medical researchers were to focus on appropriate alternatives to hysterectomy and bs-o, they could avoid technical, financial, and ethical dilemmas that artificial and transplanted ovaries and uteruses might produce.

Alternatives to Hysterectomy

The further development and use of alternatives to hysterectomy and oophorectomy is crucial. Throughout this book, I have described several possible long- and short-term problems that may be induced by gynecological surgery. In addition, it is important to recognize that some women actually die from undergoing removal of their uteruses—the overall mortality rate for elective hysterectomy is approximately 10 per 10,000. According to the RAND study (Bernstein et al. 1997), currently available alternative treatments to hysterectomy include the following:

For Leimyoma (Benign Fibroid Tumors): Myomectomy, which surgically cuts away fibroid tumors without removing the uterus; uterine artery embolization, which cuts off the blood supply to the tumors; and progesterone antagonist mifepristone (RU 486).

For Recurrent Abnormal Uterine Bleeding: Hormonal treatment; steroidal anti-inflammatory drugs; dilation and curettage (D&C); hysteroscopy with endometrial ablation; and endometrial resection by electrosurgery.

For Endometriosis: Simple extended medical observation; estrogen-progestin combinations; anti-prostaglandins; progestins; danazol; gonadotropin-releasing (GnRH) agonists; laparoscopy; excision or removal of endometrial implants through other conservative surgery; pelvic adhesion lysis; drainage and removal of endometriomas; and presacral neurectomy.

For Endometrial Hyperplasia: Dilation and curretage (D&C); medroxyprogesterone acetate (MPA).

For Pelvic Inflammatory Disease (PID): Excision or removal of pelvic abscesses; lysis of pelvic adhesions; conservative laparoscopic surgery; broad-spectrum antibiotics; pelvic rest; analgesics; and unilateral adnexectomy.

For Cervical Dysplasia: Cone biopsy; electrocagulation diathermy; cryosurgery; and laser therapy.

For Chronic Pelvic Pain: Presacral neurectomy; biofeedback, behavior modification; and stress management.

For Pelvic Relaxation and Genital Prolapse: Pelvic exercises (Kegels); pessaries; topical estrogen cream.

Of course, each of these alternative treatments has its own balance of benefits and risks, and the development of safer and more efficient alternatives must continue.

Gynecologists may not be fully aware of these alternatives, they may not be interested in learning new techniques, and performing alternatives may take longer and require more skill than hysterectomy.[4] In addition, not all insurance carriers cover alternative procedures.[5] Perhaps, if medical researchers, practitioners, and insurance companies better understood the potential significance of women's sexual reproductive organs, they might approach the problem of developing alternatives to hysterectomy and oophorectomy more aggressively.

Since any kind of surgery has the potential to disrupt identity, it is crucial that physicians ensure that patients are full "coparticipants in treatment" (Schneider and Conrad 1983, 228) by helping them to weigh positive and negative outcomes of surgery. This is especially true in the case of hysterectomy and oophorectomy. Uteruses and ovaries are potentially more relevant to an individual's sense of herself than are other body parts such as an appendix, tonsils, or gall bladder.

Recent studies conclude that women believe doctors do not spend enough time explaining issues related to menopause, hysterectomy, and hormone therapy (Galvotti and Richter 2000; Groff et al. 2000; Mingo, Herman, and Jasperse 2000). Other previous research (Allyn, Leton, Westcott et al. 1986) indicates that there is a positive correlation between degree of patient dissatisfaction with prehysterectomy counseling and later regret regarding hysterectomy. The RAND study (Bernstein et. al. 1997) argues that there are at least three distinct viewpoints with regard to the appropriateness criteria for hysterectomy: the patient, the physician, and society. Along with a detailed description of appropriate medical justifications for hysterectomy, a related RAND report, *Hysterectomy: Clinical Recommendations and Indications for Use* includes a "Cautionary Note," which states, in part:

> The expert panel felt that hysterectomy is inappropriate in all instances of benign disease if the woman desires to keep her uterus.

Finally, these recommendations do not take into account individual patient values, such as risk aversion and attitudes toward surgery. Thus, even if hysterectomy is appropriate for average (most) women with a given indication, any individual woman may appropriately opt for non-surgical therapy. (Bernstein, Kanouse, and Mittman 1997, 3)

Gynecological surgeons must take this caution more seriously and enable their patients to understand that decisions not to undergo hysterectomy or oophorectomy may be appropriate for individual women.

Feminist medical ethicists Holmes and Purdy (1992) contend that women's health care would greatly improve if physicians minimized their customary role as authorities and maximized their role as educators. Is it fair to expect gynecologists to understand the importance of gender identity? Is the moment that she is considering the possibility of surgery a propitious time for women to explore the very complicated meanings of gender identity? For many reasons, it is pleasant to envision a society in which gender identity would be completely irrelevant. Almost as pleasing is to imagine a society in which people have the opportunity to explore the meanings of gender identity throughout their lifetimes rather than at a crisis point. However, we do not yet live under those conditions. Therefore, so long as gynecologists continue to administer pap smears, deliver babies, and perform gynecological surgery, they have a responsibility to consider the complex and diverse nature of gender identity. Furthermore, they must encourage their patients to explore the subjective gender meanings that loss of bodily integrity may instigate.

Appendix

Research Methodology

FORTY-FOUR WOMEN who had experienced hysterectomies for benign conditions participated in this project. Table 2 (next page) lists the women alphabetically by pseudonym, indicating the years in which their surgeries were performed and the rationales for the surgeries. Table 3 (pages 205–209) indicates some demographic characteristics of these respondents.

I located the initial respondents through personal contacts and snowball techniques. Although I attempted to reach a more diverse sample through notices I posted in rest rooms, at colleges, and at shopping malls, I was able to locate only two respondents in this manner. I purposely did not solicit participation through either gynecologists' offices or self-help groups, since I was concerned that this might bias my sample in either a positive or negative manner. As my research progressed, I targeted specific populations, including women from lower socioeconomic classes and women who identified as bisexual or lesbian. I received several referrals from a medical clinic serving a low-income population, and I found additional bisexual and lesbian respondents by placing an advertisement in a newspaper that appeals to the gay community. Most of the respondents resided in a medium sized urban area in New England at the time they were interviewed, between 1997 and 1999.

TABLE 2 Years of and Rationales for Surgery

Name	Year of Surgery	Rationale
Alice	1987	fibroid tumors; heavy bleeding
Allison	1984	hemorrhaging (emergency)
Amber	1994	fibroid tumors, heavy bleeding
Andrea	1996	endometriosis
Anita	1977	undetermined
Ann	1994	fibroid tumors
Arlene	1988	irregular, heavy, painful periods
Barbara	1997	hemorrhaging (emergency)
Bernadette	1998	hemorrhaging during myomectomy (emergency)
Brooke	1996	fibroid tumors, continuous bleeding, polyps
Carmen	1998	complications of pregnancy
Catherine	1961	endometriosis
Charlotte	1994	hyperplasia
Christine	1985	fibroid tumors, endometriosis
Deborah	1985	fibroid tumors, hemorrhaging
Dolores	1993	vaginal bleeding
Donna	1995	endometrial hyperplasia
Ernestine	1979	enlarged uterus, scars and polyps
Esther	1964	vaginal bleeding
Ethel	1969	fibroid tumors, hemorrhaging
Faye	1986	fibroid tumors
Frances	1997	fibroid tumors
Gloria	1990	endometriosis
Isabella	1996	endometriosis, enlarged uterus
Janet	1987	endometriosis
Joy	1968	large fibroid tumor, anemia
Joyce	1989	fibroid tumors, hemorrhaging
Kelly	1997	endometriosis, heavy bleeding, pain, irregular cells
Leigh	1990	endometriosis
Letitia	1969	excessive bleeding, uterine pain
Lupe	1995	enlarged uterus
Madison	1989	endometriosis
Margie	1996	endometriosis
May	1938	heavy bleeding

TABLE 2 *Continued*

Name	Year of Surgery	Rationale
Page	hyst. and 1 ovary: 1980 2nd ovary: 1987	prolapsed uterus, ovarian cysts, endometriosis
Penny	1972	pelvic inflammatory disease
Sarah	1989	unexplained abdominal pain
Sis	1981	fibroid tumors, endometriosis
Stella	1 ovary: 1969 hyst. and 2nd ovary: 1973	abdominal infection
Sunny	1990	prolonged, heavy bleeding
Susan	1987	fibroid tumors
Terry	1984	endometriosis
Wendy	1990	scar tissue, endometriosis
Yvonne	hyst.: 1973 bs-o.: 1986	fibroid tumors irregular cells

Note: Rationales are the indications for surgery reported to me by respondents.

Of the forty-four total respondents, all of whom had hysterectomies, twenty-seven knew they had also undergone bilateral salpingo-oophorectomies (bs-o, removal of both ovaries and fallopian tubes). The two oldest respondents were not certain whether their ovaries had been removed. Three women had separate hysterectomies and oophorectomies. While the age range for all respondents was between 24 and 69, with a mean age of 38.9 years and a median age of 37.5, respondents who had undergone ovary removal ranged from 27 to 69 years of age at the time of surgery, with a mean age of 41.4 and a median age of 40. Twenty-four of these women were premenopausal prior to bilateral salpingo-oophorectomy. The rationales for respondents' oophorectomies included benign conditions such as fibroid cysts, endometriosis, adenomyosis, heavy bleeding and clotting, pelvic inflammatory disease, adhesions from previous abdominal surgery, polyps, hyperplasia, genital prolapse, unexplained pelvic discomfort, and "prophylaxis" for future risk of ovarian cancer.

Respondents chose the location of our interviews, which were usually held in their homes or at or near their workplaces. Privacy was essential, since we talked about very personal matters, and many women did not want their husbands, parents, or children to overhear us. My intent was for women to feel that the interview environment was as comfortable for them as possible, which in some cases meant that they preferred to meet in my home. In a few cases, due to geographic distance, I conducted and recorded interviews over the phone.

Interviews (ranging from 90 to 180 minutes) were open-ended and semi-structured, audio-recorded, and transcribed. I used an interview guide that was very flexible, allowing me to modify the order of questions, or even the questions themselves, depending on the specific situations of individual respondents. My interview questions also evolved as I developed better interviewing skills and as my categories of analysis became more clearly identified. At the beginning of each interview, I asked respondents to fill out a brief biographical information form. In addition to data regarding age, birthplace, marital status, and number of children, this form requested pertinent facts regarding respondents' surgeries. I found that this document provided a quick orientation to guide my questions during the interviews.

The grounded theory approach includes data analysis as an ongoing process, beginning with the initial collection of data. As the interview process progressed, I used the constant comparative method, which includes contrasting data continuously in order to explore like incidents in the development of thematic categories (Glaser and Strauss 1967). I was always alert to in vivo codes (e.g., the code words *everything* and *empty space*), and I elaborated the initial themes that arose from respondents' narratives to create more analytical themes. These form the basis for the discussion of my findings. Although my interviews were audio-recorded, I took brief field notes during each interview, which I expanded and further detailed directly afterwards. This enabled me to identify themes and issues that arose during an interview while they were still fresh in my mind. In addition, it allowed me to formulate questions that might be important to raise in subsequent interviews.

I discovered that respondents were more likely to tell me personal details about their surgeries and their lives if I first encouraged them to tell me about their backgrounds. In many cases, the most effective approach was just to let a woman talk and to pay attention while she told her story in her own way. I spent considerable time listening to stories about respondents' childhoods. Some of this, including a description of their first menstrual periods, helped me to understand how they interpreted gender identity. Tales about respondents' experiences of giving birth or attempts to get pregnant gave me insight into how they viewed their female bodies, the meaning of children in their lives, and previous gynecological and relationship issues. This initial interview stage was also important in identifying themes to probe later in the interview. Finally, some early portions of the interviews were just conversations during which the respondents and I got to know and trust each other. A number of women told me that they had never discussed their hysterectomy experiences with anyone before, including relatives, friends, and husbands. If women mentioned specific questions they wanted to ask me, I assured them that I would be happy to discuss these after the interview, which I did, with the caution that I am not a medical professional.

Some researchers criticize retrospective data because it can be distorted by imperfect memory or later events; however, this was not a problem for my project, which does not aim at discovering respondents' "true" experiences in the positivistic sense. I consider retrospective reflection an asset rather than a liability, since I sought respondents' own interpretations of the "facts," particularly in light of their subsequent life experiences.

I asked respondents both to give concrete answers to questions and to provide their own analyses. This helped me to stay as close as possible to these women's lived experiences. I was generally impressed with the insight with which women reflected on their experiences, and those respondents who were most articulate were not necessarily those who had the most education or belonged to a higher social class. In some cases, the most profound perceptions came from unexpected sources. Acknowledging the experience of the lived body allowed me to consider respondents as subjects with agency.

There are obvious drawbacks to privileging lived experience. Diana Fuss cautions that:

> Bodily experiences may seem self-evident and immediately perceptible but they are always socially mediated. Even if we were to agree that experience is not merely constructed but also itself constructing, we would still have to acknowledge that there is little agreement amongst women on exactly what constitutes "a woman's experience." Therefore we need to be extremely wary of the temptation to make substantive claims on the basis of the so-called "authority" of our experiences. (1994, 100)

I do not claim that my analysis represents the only authentic experience of hysterectomy or oophorectomy for all women in all cultures at all times. As Catherine Kohler Riessman points out, "meaning is fluid and contextual, not fixed and universal" (1993, 15). While my study may not constitute "a woman's experience," it certainly illustrates women's multiple experiences. The diversity of thoughts and feelings that forty-four women shared with me supports this.

TABLE 3 Demographic Characteristics of Respondents

Name	Bs-O?[1]	Age at Interview	Age at Surgery	Time since Surgery	Racial/ Ethnic Group	Social Class[2]	Marital Status[3]	Children	Sexual Orientation
Alice	Yes	53	43	10 yrs.	European American	Middle Class	Married	3	Hetero.
Allison	Yes	41	28	13 yrs.	European American	Middle Class	Married	2	Hetero.
Amber	Yes	42	38	4 yrs.	African American	Lower Middle Class	Single	None	Hetero.
Andrea	Yes	38	36	2 yrs.	European American	Lower Middle Class	Widow	None	Bisexual
Anita	No (1 ovary)	48	27	21 yrs.	Latina American	Working Class	Married	5	Hetero.
Ann	Yes	52	48	4 yrs.	European American	Upper Middle Class	Solemnized Union	None	Lesbian
Arlene	Yes	54	44	10 yrs.	European American	Middle Class	Divorced	2	Hetero.
Barbara	Yes	54	54	9 weeks	European American	Middle Class	Married	4	Hetero.
Bernadette	No	30	30	4 mos.	African American	Working Class	Single	None	Hetero.

(continued on next page)

TABLE 3 Continued

Name	Bs-O?[1]	Age at Interview	Age at Surgery	Time since Surgery	Racial/ Ethnic Group	Social Class[2]	Marital Status[3]	Children	Sexual Orientation
Brooke	No	36	34	2 yrs.	European American	Middle Class	Single	None	Lesbian
Carmen	No (1 ovary)	24	24	10 mos.	Latina American	Lower Class	Single	3	Hetero.
Catherine	Yes	69	32	37 yrs.	European American	Upper Middle Class	Divorced (Married)	5	Hetero.
Charlotte	Yes (2 surgeries)	56	52	4 yrs.	European American	Working Class	Married	None	Hetero.
Christine	No (piece left)	51	38	13 yrs.	European American	Lower Middle Class	Annulled	None	Lesbian (hetero. at time)
Deborah	Yes	77	65	12 yrs.	European American	Middle Class	Married	2	Hetero.
Dolores	Yes	74	69	5 yrs.	Latina American	Lower Class	Married	18	Hetero.
Donna	No	40	37	3 yrs.	European American	Working Class	Married	None	Hetero.
Ernestine	No	59	40	19 yrs.	European American	Working Class	Divorced (Married)	4	Hetero.

Name	Bs-O?[1]	Age at Interview	Age at Surgery	Time since Surgery	Racial/ Ethnic Group	Social Class[2]	Marital Status[3]	Children	Sexual Orientation
Esther	Doesn't Know	84	51	33 yrs.	European American	Middle Class	Married	1	Hetero.
Ethel	Yes	74	46	28 yrs.	European American	Middle Class	Married	2	Hetero.
Faye	No (1 ovary)	56	44	12 yrs.	African American	Upper Middle Class	Divorced	1	Hetero.
Frances	Yes	50	49	1 yr.	European American	Upper Middle Class	Divorced	None	Hetero.
Gloria	No (1 ovary)	47	39	8 yrs.	European American	Working Class	Single	None	Lesbian
Isabella	Yes	39	37	2 yrs.	Latina American	Lower Class	Partnered	2	Hetero.
Janet	Yes	49	39	10 yrs.	European American	Middle Class	Divorced (Married)	3	Hetero.
Joy	No	65	35	30 yrs.	European American	Upper Middle Class	Married	3	Hetero.
Joyce	No	49	41	8 yrs.	European American	Upper Middle Class	Divorced (Married)	2	Hetero.

(continued on next page)

TABLE 3 Continued

Name	Bs-O?[1]	Age at Interview	Age at Surgery	Time since Surgery	Racial/ Ethnic Group	Social Class[2]	Marital Status[3]	Children	Sexual Orientation
Kelly	Yes	46	45	1 year	European American	Middle Class	Married	2	Hetero.
Leigh	Yes	43	34	9 yrs.	European American	Middle Class	Married	None	Hetero.
Letitia	Yes	56	27	29 yrs.	European American	Working Class	Divorced (Married)	3	Hetero.
Lupe	No	34	31	3 yrs.	Latina American	Middle Class	Married	2	Hetero.
Madison	Yes	48	39	9 yrs.	European American	Upper Middle Class	Married	2	Hetero.
Margie	Yes	35	33	2 yrs.	European American	Middle Class	Single	None	Bisexual
May	Doesn't Know	97	37	60 yrs.	European American	Middle Class	Widowed (Married)	None	Hetero.
Page	Yes 2 surgeries	51	hyst. and 1st ovary: 33; 2nd ovary: 40	hyst: 18; 2nd ovary: 11	European American	Upper Middle Class	Married	3	Hetero.
Penny	No	53	27	26 yrs.	European American	Working Class	Married	None	Hetero.

Name	Bs-O?[1]	Age at Interview	Age at Surgery	Time since Surgery	Racial/ Ethnic Group	Social Class[2]	Marital Status[3]	Children	Sexual Orientation
Sarah	Yes	49	40	9 yrs.	European American	Middle Class	Married	2	Hetero.
Sis	Yes	47	28	19 yrs.	European American	Lower Middle Class	Married (Divorced)	None	Hetero.
Stella	Yes 2 surgeries	56	1 ovary: 27; hyst. and 2nd ovary: 31	1 ovary: 29; hyst. and 2nd ovary: 25	European American	Lower Class	Divorced	3	Hetero.
Sunny	Yes	48	41	7 yrs.	European American	Middle Class	Married	1 (3 step)	Hetero.
Susan	No	52	41	11 yrs.	European American	Upper Middle Class	Married	None	Hetero.
Terry	Yes	47	33	14 yrs.	European American	Upper Middle Class	Divorced (Married)	2 (adopted)	Hetero.
Wendy	No (1 ovary)	42	34	8 yrs.	European American	Homeless	Divorced	2	Hetero.
Yvonne	Yes 2 surgeries	61	hyst.: 37 bs-o.: 49	hyst.: 24 bs-o.: 12	European American	Middle Class	Married	2	Hetero.

[1]Bilateral salpingo-oophorectomy (surgical removal of both fallopian tubes and both ovaries).

[2]Social class is by self-report.

[3]First listing indicates marital status at time of interview; second listing indicates marital status at time of surgery.

Notes

Chapter 1

Epigraph: From Anne Sexton, "In Celebration of My Uterus," *Love Poems* (Boston: Houghton Mifflin, 1969).

1. *Microsoft Encarta 97 Encyclopedia* includes the following inaccurate statement under the definition of hysterectomy: "Sometimes only the uterus and cervix are removed; in other cases, called a complete hysterectomy, the uterus, cervix, fallopian tubes, and ovaries are all removed."

2. See the Postscript for further discussion.

3. Another surgical procedure performed only on women, cesarean section, is now the most common of all surgical procedures.

4. The average age of American women undergoing hysterectomy is 42.7 and the median age is 40.9. By contrast, natural menopause is completed over several years, with the last menstrual period occurring at an average age of 51 for American women (ACOG 1992b).

5. Barbara Ehrenreich and Deirdre English (1978) refer to the Victorian theory that women's "natural" characteristics were directly attributable to their ovaries as the "psychology of the ovary."

6. Angier (1999) explains that female ovaries correspond to male testes, the female analogue of the male penis is the clitoris, and the female labia are the structural counterpart to the scrotum; "the uterus alone offers a clear case of presence versus absence" (84).

7. Some illustrations of the use of uteruses or ovaries to represent women are: "Women owe their manner of being to their organs of generation and especially to the uterus" (Dr. Claude Martin Gardien, 1816, quoted in Laqueur 1990, 149); "It is only because of the ovary that a woman is what she is" (Dr. Achille Chéreau, 1844, qtd. in Laqueur 1990,

175); "The ovaries give to woman all her characteristics of body and mind. We need not explain how or why" (Dr. George L. Austin, 1873, qtd. in Corea 1977, 92; "The active or dominant organ of the sexual system is the ovary" (Doctors Robert and Fancourt Barnes, 1884, qtd. in Mosucci 1990, 34); "A woman exists only through her ovaries" (Victor Jozé, 1885, qtd. in Laqueur 1990, 14); "It was as if the Almighty, in creating the female sex, had taken the uterus and built up a woman around it" (nineteenth-century physician, qtd. in Rosenberg 1975, 335).

8. Medical sociologists who have researched this include Bury (1982); Charmaz (1983; 1991; 1994); Corbin and Strauss (1987); Greil (1991a, 1991b); Karp (1999); Murphy (1999); Schneider and Conrad (1983); Strauss et al. (1984).

9. Although the physicians who first attempted abdominal surgery were widely applauded for their courage and competence, the early women who endured ovariotomy (without the benefit of anesthesia) were not recognized as important pioneers.

10. Toward the end of the twentieth century, it again became a more frequent practice to surgically remove uteruses vaginally, often with laparoscopic assistance, which is a less invasive procedure than abdominal surgery.

11. See Elson 1996, 2000, 2001a,b,c; 2002. The earliest sociological study I was able to find on this topic was a 51-page 1959 dissertation (Hawkinson 1959) that focused on the impact of women's hysterectomies on significant others rather than on women as subjects.

12. Some researchers who came to this conclusion include Ananth (1978); Barker (1968); Chynoweth and Abrahams (1977); Darling and McKoy-Smith (1993); Derogatis (1980); Drelich and Bieber (1958); Kav-Venaki and Zakham (1983); Martin, Roberts, and Clayton (1980); Melody (1962); Nadelson, Notman, and Ellis (1983); Palmer (1984); Raphael (1972); D. H. Richards (1973, 1974); and Schumaker (1990).

13. Including studies by Cosper, Fuller, and Robinson (1978); Everson et al. (1995), Hampton and Tarnasky (1974); Harris (1997); Patterson and Craig (1963); B.C. Richards (1978); and Stein (1991).

14. This includes studies by Ackner (1960); Carlson (1997); Gath et al. (1995); Lalinec-Michaud and Englesman (1984); and Webb and Wilson-Barnett (1983).

15. This research includes studies by Ackner (1960); Cooper, and Day (1982); Gath, Ryan, Dennerstein, and Pepperell (1989); Melody (1962); McKinlay, McKinlay, and Brambilla (1987); and Moore and Tolley (1976).

16. This parallels a study by Reinharz (1987) of self-help books regarding miscarriage.

17. For a previous project (Elson 1996), I reviewed the following self-help books: *The No-Hysterectomy Option: Your Body—Your Choice* (Gold-

farb 1990); *No More Hysterectomies* (Hufnagel 1989); *Coping with a Hysterectomy: Your Choice, Your Own Solutions* (Morgan 1982); *How to Avoid a Hysterectomy: An Indispensable Guide to Exploring All Your Options Before You Consent to a Hysterectomy* (Payer 1987); *Male Practice: How Doctors Manipulate Women* (Mendelsohn 1981); *You Don't Need a Hysterectomy: New and Effective Ways of Avoiding Major Surgery* (Strausz 1993); *The Hysterectomy Hoax* (West 1994); *Hysterectomy: Learning the Facts, Coping with the Feelings, Facing the Future* (Williams 1982); *Hysterectomy: Before and After* (Cutler 1990); *Recovering from a Hysterectomy* (Harris and MacLean 1992); *The Castrated Woman: What Your Doctor Won't Tell You About Hysterectomy* (Stokes 1986). In addition, in preparation for this book I reviewed additional self-help volumes, including *Our Bodies Ourselves for the New Century* (Boston Women's Health Book Collective 1998); *Just as Much a Woman: Your Personal Guide to Hysterectomy and Beyond* (Rosenfeld and Bolen 1999); *The Premature Menopause Book: When the Change Comes Too Early* (Petras 1999); and *The Ultimate Rape: What Every Woman Should Know About Hysterectomies and Ovarian Removal* (Plourde 1998).

18. Hyster Sisters Web site (www.hystersisters.com), retrieved June 2002. Some narratives on the Hyster Sisters Web site are more bizarre than others, with one ending: "The King looked down and saw the love and unity of the Princesses and knew that the book was in good hands and smiled. He could see that all was well in the land of Hyster and Waiting and that all was hormonally balanced!!" There is also an online Hyster Sister store offering such goodies as T-shirts, night shirts, mouse pads, pillows, mugs, and note cards as well as dolls called "Hilda Hotflash," "Ester-Jenn," and "Insomnia Sue," and an adjustable crown in order to "make sure family and friends remember to pamper the princess."

19. For example, Susanne Morgan, the author of *Coping with a Hysterectomy* (1982), happens to be a medical sociologist. However, her book presents a political self-help discourse, rather than a sociological text.

20. This includes research by Bernhard 1985; 1992; Chasse 1990; Dell 2000; Dell and Papagiannidou 1999; Kinnick and Leners 1995; Krull 2000; Ryan 1997; and Webb and Wilson-Barnett 1983. In addition, since I completed my original study, initial results of the Ethnicity, Needs, and Decisions of Women at Midlife (ENDOW) Project (Richter and Galavotti 2000) were released. This study was funded by the Centers Disease Control and Prevention (CDC) Division of Reproductive Health and the National Institutes of Health (NIH) Women Health Initiative (WHI). The ENDOW project focused on how women of various ethnicities made decisions regarding hysterectomy, surgical menopause, and the use of hormone replacement therapy (HRT). Although primarily a quantitative study, focus group discussions and interviews were used in the initial phase of the ENDOW project in order to develop survey instru-

ments. The initial qualitative results were released in a special issue of the *Journal of Women's Health and Gender-Based Medicine*. Qualitative techniques will also be use to guide intervention development (Richter and Galavotti 2000).

Chapter 2

Acknowledgments: A version of this chapter will appear as an article, "Hormonal Hierarchy: Hysterectomy and Stratified Stigma," in *Gender & Society* (forthcoming). Earlier versions were presented at the American Sociological Association and the Eastern Sociological Society in 2001.

Epigraphs: From Susan Wendell, *The Rejected Body: Feminist Philosophical Reflections on Disability* (New York: Routledge, 1996), and from Susan Bordo, *Unbearable Weight: Feminism, Western Culture and the Body* (Berkeley: University of California Press, 1993).

1. The two oldest respondents were not certain whether their ovaries had been removed. Three women had separate surgeries: an earlier hysterectomy and a later bilateral salpingo-oophorectomy.

2. By contrast, considerable debate has surrounded state laws involving either mandatory or voluntary chemical (reversible) castration of male sex offenders. Opponents, including the ACLU, have asserted that chemical castration violates the Eighth Amendment prohibition against "cruel and unusual punishment." Psychologists and Psychiatrists have testified to the emotional harm caused even by temporary chemical castration (Jenkins 1998).

3. Hufnagel proposes that ovarian failure probably occurs because "the massive dissection occurring during a hysterectomy interrupts a great deal of the blood supply to the ovaries of many women" (Hufnagel 1989, 26). In addition, there is medical speculation that in order to ovulate; the ovaries may require stimulation of prostaglandins found in the uterus (Siddle, Sarrel, and Whitehead 1987).

4. Ovaries measure approximately 1 by 1.5 inches.

Chapter 3

Acknowledgment: An earlier version of this chapter received the 1999 Graduate Student Paper Award from the Health, Health Policy, and Health Services Division of the Society for the Study of Social Problems.

Epigraph: From Peter Conrad, "The Meaning of Medications: Another Look at Compliance," *Social Science and Medicine* 20:29–37, 1985.

1. Small quantities of these hormones are produced in the adrenal glands, and androgens are converted to estrogen by fat tissue, as well (NWHN 2002, 35).

2. See Berek 1996; Boston Women's Health Book Collective 1994; 1998; Hufnagel 1989; Love with Lindsey 1998; Rock and Thompson 1997.

3. For example, compare ACOG 1992c with National Women's Health Network 1995.

4. Anthropologist Margaret Mead was probably the first to claim that many women experience renewed energy following menopause: "There is no greater power than the zest of a postmenopausal woman" (qtd. in Sheehy 1993, 118).

5. The terms ET (to indicate estrogen therapy, rather than ERT) and CHT (combined hormone therapy, instead of HRT) are used in "The Menopause, Hormone Therapy, and Women's Health," published by the US Congress Office of Technology Assessment (1992) in order to acknowledge that natural menopause does not cause an estrogen deficiency that requires replacement. This language is not yet in general use.

6. These include Boston Women's Health Book Collective 1998; Coney 1994; Doress-Waters and Siegal 1994; Greenwood 1996; Ito 1994; Love with Lindsey 1998; Ojeda 1992; Taylor and Sumrall 1991; Weed 1991).

7. At the 1993 meeting of a professional conference, one of the sessions included a discussion of how unnecessary exogenous hormones are "pushed" on menopausal women. The discussion leader attempted to prove this point by passing around glossy brochures published by pharmaceutical companies to promote the sale of hormone therapy. She explained to the group that these brochures were deceptive because they featured pictures of young women to advertise their products, while the potential menopausal customers are considerably older. I suggested that maybe these younger women were the *appropriate* target consumers for hormone therapy since they might have experienced surgical menopause.

8. Interestingly, Martin (1992) found that, while younger women in her study anticipated natural menopause as a time when bodies go out of control, women past natural menopause did not describe their experiences in this way.

9. Besides through bilateral oophorectomy, women may reach premature menopause naturally or through chemotherapy or radiation treatments.

10. An indication of this cultural belief in the power of hormones to determine appropriate gender behavior is the following news story. In an

obvious attempt at insult, California Congressional candidate Bob Dornan "asserted that one of his GOP primary opponents, wealthy divorce lawyer Lisa Hughes, who [was] waging an aggressive campaign against him, 'has more testosterone than estrogen'" (Benedetto 1998).

11. A recent advertising slogan emphasizes the connection to natural estrogen: "Premarin will continue to be *my estrogen*, now more than ever." [Emphasis mine]

12. There are inconsistent findings regarding the effects of soy or genistein on human bone density, and "One consistent finding is that soy, unlike estrogen, does not reduce oophorectomy-induced bone turnover" (National Women's Health Network 2002, 89).

13. Medical researchers have just recently begun to successfully reimplant pieces of ovaries into the abdomens of women from whom they were removed and frozen when younger (Weiss 1999). Transplantation of ovaries was previously attempted at the beginning of the twentieth century (Squier 2000).

14. Including Berek (1996, 151–5); Rock and Thompson (1997, 995–7).

15. ACOG (1992a,b).

16. For example, Boston Women's Health Book Collective 1998; Col 1997; Coney 1994; Doress-Waters and Siegal 1994; Dranov 1993; Greer 1992; Jacobowitz 1993; Lark 1995; Love with Lindsey1998; Montreal Health Press 1997; National Women's Health Network 1995; Sheehy 1992; Utian and Jacobowitz 1990; and Voda 1997.

17. Kaufert and McKinlay (1985, 125) report: "Whether one views the role of the press in positive or negative terms, the publicity had a major responsibility for the reduction in the use of estrogen after 1975. . . . Media publicity served to carry the message of the researcher—that estrogen was potentially iatrogenic—into the wider medical community and to the lay public, including women taking estrogen."

18. The final report of the 1979 Consensus Development Conference on Estrogen Use and Post-Menopausal Women, sponsored by the National Institute on Aging, concluded that ERT "should be administered on a cyclical basis (3 weeks on, 1 week off), at the lowest dose for the shortest possible time" (qtd. in McCrea 1983, 115).

19. According to Kolata (2002): "The data indicate that if 10,000 women take the drugs for a year, 8 more will develop invasive breast cancer as compared with 10,000 women who were not taking hormone replacement therapy. An additional 7 will have a heart attack, 8 will have a stroke, and 18 will have blood clots. But there will be 6 fewer colorectal cancers and 5 fewer hip fractures."

20. In May 2003, it was announced that the Women's Heath Initiative Memory Study (WHIMS) had determined that estrogen plus progestin therapy actually increased the risk for probable dementia in post-

menopausal women 65 or older. In addition, HRT did not prevent mild cognitive impairment in these women (Shumaker, Legault, and Thal et al. 2003).

21. Prior to the results of the HERS and WHI studies, several observational studies indicated that ERT might have a protective effect on the heart. However, "Studies have found that ERT users are less likely to smoke and to have diabetes and are more physically active and leaner. . . . Also, women who take ERT are more likely to make lifestyle changes that lower the risk of disease than are other women of the same social and economic group. Moreover, health care providers may be less likely to prescribe estrogen to women who have higher risk of heart disease" (NWHN 2002, 179).

22. Uncertainty has long been recognized as part of the experience of illness (e.g., Bury 1982; Conrad 1987; Corbin and Strauss 1987; Davis 1960; Fox 1957; Greil 1991a; 1991b; Mechanic 1968; Parsons 1951; Roth 1963).

Chapter 4

Acknowledgments: An earlier version of this chapter appeared as an article, "Menarche, menstruation, and gender identity: Retrospective accounts from women who have undergone premenopausal hysterectomy," *Sex Roles* 46 (1/2) (January 2002). A still earlier version was presented at the June 2001 meeting of the Society for Menstrual Cycle Research in Avon, Connecticut.

Epigraph: From J. P. Greenhill, *Office Gynecology,* 6th ed., quoted in Lander (1988, 65).

1. Angier (1999) had several conversations with people born with *androgenital syndrome* (AGS). These individuals each have an X and Y chromosome (which would make them genetically male), but they also have defective androgen receptors, which cause them to develop the secondary sexual characteristics of females. Thus, they are generally brought up and treated as women. "Interestingly," Angier found, "many of them say the thing they regret most is not their inability to have children but the lack of menstruation, the event they see as a *monthly voucher of femaleness*" (p. 33; emphasis added).

2. The 1977 establishment of the Society for Menstrual Cycle Research, which promotes woman-centered research on menstruation, is a case in point.

3. Delaney, Lupton, and Toth have pointed out, however, that "although most men do not bleed from their genitals every month as women do, men's behavior does follow distinct cycles" and that all humans are

"subject to *circadian*, or 24-hour cycles: a flux in hormones, moods, strengths, and weaknesses" (1976, 267). In like manner, Lander comments, "It is not women who are cyclic, it is all of us, and all of us ignore our cyclicity at our peril" (1988, 145).

Chapter 5

Epigraphs: From Edward Carpenter, "Woman in Freedom," in *Loves Coming of Age* (New York and London: Mitchell Kennerley, 1911), and from Patricia A. Kaufert, "Myth and the Menopause," *Sociology of Health and Illness* 4 (2): 141–66, July 1982.

1. Althaus (cited in Shinberg 1998), among other researchers, finds that women who have had tubal sterilizations are more likely to undergo hysterectomy than other women, particularly in the years immediately following their sterilizations.

2. Although Margie described herself as bisexual, she prefers to call herself "sexual" because she doesn't "relate to labels."

3. I met one of my respondents due to a similar statement I made regarding the use of the term "childbearing years" by members of a women's health collective who were giving a presentation at a professional conference. Donna publicly thanked me for making the statement, later told me she had had a hysterectomy, and agreed to be interviewed.

4. In fall of 1999 it was widely reported, including by the *Boston Globe* (Weiss 1999) and *The New York Times* (Stolberg 1999), that for the first time doctors were able to restore fertility in a thirty-year-old ballerina by reimplanting into her abdomen several pieces of her ovaries that had been removed and frozen when she was younger. This procedure could possibly allow postmenopausal women to become pregnant. However, since respondents in my study have all had hysterectomies, they no longer have uteruses, and so would be unable to carry a fetus regardless of the status of their ovaries. Attempts to transplant uteruses and to create artificial uteruses are discussed in the Postscript.

5. Bernadette was referring to an assisted fertility procedure known as gestational surrogacy, whereby a woman is able to contract to have her biological child implanted in the uterus of another woman.

6. Drellich and Bieber (1958) found that it was common for women who had hysterectomies to complain of excessive appetite, overeating, and weight gain in the postoperative period, which they suggest may have been caused by attempts to fill up the void created by the missing uterus.

7. A pessary is a rubber device that is sometimes used to prop up internal organs and thus avoid surgery. The pessary usually fits around the cervix (the neck of the womb). Since Catherine's cervix was removed

when she had a hysterectomy, it is logical that she had difficulty retaining pessaries.

Chapter 6

Epigraphs: From Robert J. Stoller, *Sex and Gender,* Vol. 1, *The Development of Masculinity and Femininity* (New York: Jason Aronson, 1968), and from Shania Twain and Robert John Lange, "Man! I Feel Like a Woman!" *Come on Over* (New York: Mercury Records, 1997).

1. Brooks-Gunn and Kirsch 1984; Greer 1992; Lee and Sasser-Coen 1996; Ussher 1989.

2. Wukasch (1996) determined that women with a history of rape and/or incest had significantly higher levels of depression the first year after hysterectomy than women who had not been abused. In addition, Hendricks-Matthews (1991) found that gynecological surgery may reawaken the earlier traumatic experiences of women who have been sexually abused.

3. Interestingly, although much contemporary medical discourse denies that women might have lessened sexual desire and decreased ability to enjoy sex after gynecological surgery, nineteenth- and early-twentieth-century medical discourse promoted it as a cure for nymphomania: "Orgasm was the disease, and the cure was orgasm's destruction" (qtd. in Barker-Benfield 1977, 32). The absence of sexual desire was considered an important feminine quality for Victorian women. Even as late as the early to mid-twentieth century, "female sexuality, including female orgasm, was understood as being in the service of greater male satisfaction, both psychological and sexual" (Schneider and Gould 1987, 126; see also Miller and Fowlkes 1980).

4. For example, Puretz and Haas (1993) compared sexual desire and responsiveness based upon self-reports and found no differences between premenopausal women and those who had undergone either natural menopause or hysterectomy. However, these researchers did not specifically distinguish between hysterectomized women who had bs-o and those who did not.

5. In their review of studies regarding the effect of oophorectomy on sexual behavior, Ford and Beach (1952, quoted in Drelich and Bieber 1958, 327) found that women were capable of both feeling sexual desire and successfully participating in sexual acts regardless of whether their ovaries had been removed. They conclude, "Ovariectomy and the advent of surgical menopause in mature females does not in itself necessarily cause a decrease in sexual desire or capabilities" (327). Unfortunately, no mention is made of whether women were taking any form of hormone replacement therapy.

6. This includes research conducted by Bachmann 1990; Guzick and Hoeger 2000; Sherwin and Gelfand 1987; Sherwin, Gelfand, and Brender 1985; Stoller 1968.

7. It is important to note that, according to Thomas G. Stovall, Professor of obstetrics and gynecology at the University of Tennessee at Memphis, "The positive results from the Maryland study indicate the patients who were followed had been properly selected and really needed the surgery" (Gentry 1999). The Maryland researchers caution that their data should not be interpreted to indicate that the removal of a healthy uterus would improve sexual functioning.

Chapter 7

Epigraphs: From Juliet Corbin and Anselm L. Strauss, "Accompaniments of Chronic Illness: Changes in Body, Self, Biography, and Biographical Time," pp. 249–81 in Julius Roth and Peter Conrad, eds., *The Experience and Management of Chronic Illness: Research in the Sociology of Health Care,* Vol. 6 (Greenwich, CT: JAI Press, 1987), and from Judith A. Howard and Jocelyn Hollander, *Gendered Situations, Gendered Selves: A Gender Lens on Social Psychology* (Walnut Creek, CA: Altamira Press, 1997).

1. This includes research done by Bernhard 1985; Cosper, Fuller, and Robinson 1978; Keith 1980; Morgan 1982; Roopnarinesingh and Gopeesingh 1982.

2. This includes studies conducted by Bernhard 1992; Chynoweth and Abrahams 1977; Jackson 1992; Jordan 2002; Newman and Newman 1985; Raphael 1978; Roeske 1978; Rosenhand 1984; Smith and Reilly 1994; Webb and Wilson-Barnett 1983.

3. Andrea told me that her partner at the time was a man who "always wanted to be a woman."

Chapter 8

Epigraphs: From Natalie Angier, *Woman: An Intimate Geography* (Boston: Houghton Mifflin, 1999), and from Susan Bordo, *Unbearable Weight: Feminism, Western Culture and the Body* (Berkeley: University of California Press, 1993).

1. I cannot resist the temptation to speculate whether that means that hermaphrodite people occupy "extra-liminal" space while hysterectomized people occupy "sub-liminal" space.

2. An attempt at framing hysterectomy from a postmodern perspective was attempted following my original study (Dell 2000). However,

the researcher draws only on interviews with ten middle-class women who lived in traditional families in Greece, were middle aged, and had generally completed childbearing.

3. Bush (1999, 442) makes a similar, though not identical, argument when she points out that, "to participate in cervical screening, individuals must have a cervix, they must be, biologically and anatomically female."

4. A "laparoscopy" entails the examination of the abdominal cavity by the insertion of a lighted, hollow metal instrument, called a "laparoscope."

5. It is important to note that "emergency hysterectomy, a situation where preoperative counseling is curtailed, is associated with a higher incidence of psychological problems than are elective procedures," according to Bachmann (1990, 43).

6. Another helpful analogy, developed by Marcel Mauss (1979), is described in Turner 1992). Mauss claims that fundamental aspects of embodied human activity, such as walking, standing, or sitting require a common organic foundation, but also become uniquely influenced by cultural and personal differences.

Postscript

1. This research includes findings that women are more likely to undergo hysterectomies if they are African American, on welfare, receive Medicaid, are unwed mothers, have had multiple abortions, have low educational attainment, lack vocational training, or reside in communities with lower than average income levels.

2. This procedure was performed because the Saudi woman wanted to have another child and Islamic law does not allow the use of surrogate mothers because it is forbidden for genetic coding (including eggs and embryos) to be transferred from one person to another. However, uterus transplants were deemed permissible.

3. A Japanese medical researcher has apparently succeeded in keeping goat fetuses that have been nurtured in artificial wombs alive up to several weeks (Cook 2002).

4. In discussing alternatives to hysterectomy, Michael Broder, assistant professor of obstetrics and gynecology at UCLA states, "Medicine is a very conservative field and tends not to move unless it's shoved" (quoted in Shari Roan, "Despite options, hysterectomy rates unchanged," *Keene (N.H.) Sentinel,* 28 March 2002, 13).

5. See Elizabeth Cooney, "An alternative to hysterectomy," *Worcester* (Mass.) *Telegram and Gazette,* 11 March 2002, C1, C3.

References

Ackner, B. 1960. "Emotional aspects of hysterectomy: A follow-up study of fifty patients under the age of forty." Pp. 248–52 in A. Jores and H. Freyberger (eds.), *Advances in Psychosomatic Medicine*. New York: Brunner.

Allgeier, E. R., and A. R. Allgeier. 1991. *Sexual interactions*, 3rd ed. Lexington, MA: D. C. Heath.

Allsworth, J. E., S. Zierler, N. Krieger, B. L. Harlow. 2001. "Ovarian function in late reproductive years in relation to lifetime experiences of abuse." *Epidemiology* 12 (6) (November): 676–81.

Allyn, D. P., D. A. Leton, N. A. Westcott, et al. 1986. "Presterilization counseling and women's regret about having been sterilized." *Journal of Reproductive Medicine* 31 (11): 1027–32.

American College of Obstetricians and Gynecologists [ACOG] Patient Education. 1992a. *Understanding hysterectomy*. Washington, DC: American College of Obstetricians and Gynecologists.

———. 1992b. *The menopause years*. Washington, DC: American College of Obstetricians and Gynecologists.

———. 1992c. *Hormone replacement therapy*. Washington, DC: American College of Obstetricians and Gynecologists.

Ananth, J. 1978. "Hysterectomy and Depression." *Obstetrics and Gynecology* 2 (6): 727–33.

———. 1983. "Hysterectomy and sexual counseling." *Psychiatric Journal of the University of Ottawa* 8: 213–17.

Angier, Natalie. 1997. "In culture of hysterectomies, many question their necessity." *New York Times*, February 17, A1.

———. 1999. *Woman: An intimate geography*. Boston: Houghton Mifflin.

Annegers, J. F., H. Strom, D. G. Decker, M. B. Dockerty, and M. O'Fallon. 1979. "Ovarian cancer: Incidence and case-control study." *Cancer* 43: 723–29.

Bachmann, Gloria A. 1990. "Psychosexual aspects of hysterectomy." *Women's Health Issues* 1: 41–49.

Barker, Montague G. 1968. "Psychiatric illness after hysterectomy." *British Medical Journal* 2 (April): 91–95.

Barker-Benfield, G. J. 1976. *The horrors of the half-known life: Male attitudes toward women and sexuality in nineteenth-century America.* New York: Harper and Row.

Bartky, Sandra Lee. 1998 [1992]. "Foucault, femininity, and the modernization of patriarchal power." Pp. 25–45 in Rose Weitz, ed., *The politics of women's bodies: Sexuality, appearance, and behavior.* New York: Oxford University Press.

Beavis, E. L. G., J. B. Brown, M. A. Smith. 1969. "Ovarian function after hysterectomy with conservation of the ovaries in premenopausal women." *Journal of Obstetrics and Gynaecology, British Commonwealth* 76: 969.

Becker, Gay. 1994. "Metaphors in disrupted lives: Infertility and cultural constructions of continuity." *Medical Anthropology Quarterly* (new series) 8 (4) (December): 383–410.

Bell, Susan. 1987. "Changing ideas: The medicalization of menopause." *Social Science and Medicine* 24: 525–42.

Bellerose, Satya B. 1989. "Body image and sexuality in surgically menopausal women." Ph.D. diss., McGill University.

Bellerose, S. B., and Y. M. Binik. 1993. "Body image and sexuality in oophorectomized women." *Archives of Sexual Behavior* 22: 435–59.

Berek, Jonathan S., ed. 1996. *Novak's gynecology.* Baltimore: Williams and Wilkins.

Bernhard, Linda A. 1985. "Black women's concerns about sexuality and hysterectomy." *Sage: A Scholarly Journal on Black Women* 2 (2): 25–27.

———. 1986. "Methodology issues in studies of sexuality and hysterectomy." *Journal of Sex Research* 22 (1) (February): 108–28.

———. 1992. "Consequences of hysterectomy in the lives of women." *Health Care for Women International* 13: 281.

Bernhard, L. A., C. R. Harris, and H. A. Caroline. 1992. "Men's views about hysterectomies and the women who have them." *Image: Journal of Nursing Scholarship* 24 (3) (fall): 177–81.

———. 1997. "Partner communication about hysterectomy." *Health Care for Women International* 18: 73–83.

Bernstein, Steven J., Mary E. Fisk, Elizabeth A. McGlynn, and Diedre S. Gifford. 1997. *Hysterectomy: A review of the literature on indications, effectiveness, and risks.* Santa Monica, CA: RAND.

Bernstein, Steven J., David E. Kanouse, and Brian S. Mitman. 1997. *Hysterectomy: Clinical recommendations and indications for use.* Santa Monica, CA: RAND.

Bleier, Ruth. 1984. *Science and gender: A critique of biology and its theories on women.* Oxford: Pergamon Press.

Block Lewis, Helen. 1976. *Psychic war in men and women.* New York: New York University Press.

Blumstein, Philip W. 1975. "Identity bargaining and self-conception." *Social Forces* 53 (3) (March): 476–85.

Bordo, Susan. 1993. *Unbearable weight: Feminism, Western culture and the body.* Berkeley: University of California Press.

Boston Women's Health Book Collective (BWHBC). 1992. *The new our bodies ourselves.* New York: Simon and Schuster.

————. 1998. *Our bodies ourselves for the new century.* New York: Simon and Schuster.

Brody, Jane. 1993. "A decline in hysterectomy still falls short." *New York Times,* June 30, C14.

Brooks-Gunn, Jeanne, and Barbara Kirsch. 1984. "Life events and the boundaries of midlife for women." Pp. 31–68 in Grace Baruch and Jeanne Brooks-Gunn, eds., *Women in midlife.* New York: Basic Books.

Broverman, Inge, Susan Vogel, Donald Broverman, Frank Clarkson, and Paul Rosenkrantz. 1972. "Sex role stereotypes: A current appraisal." *Journal of Social Issues* 28: 59–78.

Brownmiller, Susan. 1984. *Femininity.* New York: Fawcett Columbine.

Bury, Michael. 1982. "Chronic illness as biographical disruption." *Sociology of Health and Illness* 4 (2) (July): 167–82.

Bush, Judith. 1999. "'It's just part of being a woman'": Cervical screening, the body and femininity." *Social Science and Medicine* 50: 429–44.

Butler, Judith. 1990. *Gender trouble: Feminism and the subversion of identity.* New York and London: Routledge.

————. 1993. *Bodies that matter.* New York and London: Routledge.

Callahan, Joan C. 1993. *Menopause: A midlife passage.* Bloomington: Indiana University Press.

Carlson, K. J. 1997. "Outcomes of hysterectomy." *Clinical Obstetrics and Gynecology* 40 (4) (December): 939–46.

Carlson, Karen J., David H. Nichols, and Isaac Schiff. 1993. "Indications for hysterectomy." *New England Journal of Medicine* 328 (12) (March 25): 856.

Carpenter, Edward. 1911. "Woman in Freedom." In *Loves coming of age.* New York and London: Mitchell Kennerley.

Cauley, J. A., S. R. Cummings, D. M. Black, S. R. Mascioli, and D. G. Seeley. 1990. "Prevalence and determinants of estrogen replacement therapy in elderly women." *American Journal of Obstetrics and Gynecology* 165: 1438–40.

Charmaz, Kathy. 1983. "Loss of self: A fundamental form of suffering in the chronically ill." *Sociology of Health and Illness* 5 (2): 168–95.

226   References

————. 1991. *Good days, bad days: The self in chronic illness and time.* New Brunswick, NJ: Rutgers University Press.

————. 1994. "Discoveries of self in illness." Pp. 226–42 in Mary Lorenz Dietz, Robert Prus, and William Shaffir, eds., *Doing everyday life: Ethnography as human lived Experience.* Toronto: Copp Clark Longman Ltd.

————. 1999a. "Discoveries of self in illness." Pp. 72–81 in Kathy Charmaz and Debora A. Paterniti, eds., *Health, illness, and healing: Society, social context and self: An anthology.* Los Angeles: Roxbury.

————. 1999b. "The body, identity, and self: Adapting to impairment." Pp. 95–112 in Kathy Charmaz and Debora A. Paterniti, eds., *Health, illness, and healing: Society, social context and self: An anthology.* Los Angeles: Roxbury.

Chasse, Marie-Andree. 1990. *The experiences of women who undergo hysterectomy.* Master's thesis, University of Alberta.

Chodorow, Nancy. 1978. *The reproduction of mothering: Psychoanalysis and the sociology of gender.* Berkeley: University of California Press.

Chodorow, Nancy, and Susan Contratto. 1982. "The fantasy of the perfect mother." Pp. 54–75 in Barrie Thorne and Marilyn Yalom, eds., *Rethinking the family: Some feminist questions.* New York: Longman.

Chynoweth, R., and M. J. Abrahams. 1977. "Psychological complications of hysterectomy." *Australian and New Zealand Journal of Obstetrics and Gynaecology* 17: 40–44. [Cited in Carol Stein (1991), "The relationship of hysterectomy surgery and self-perception of femininity to mood and sexual satisfaction," Ph.D. diss., California School of Professional Psychology.]

Col, Nananda Francette. 1997. *A woman doctor's guide to hormone therapy.* Worcester, MA: Tatnuck Bookseller Press.

Coltrane, Scott. 1989. "Household labor and the routine production of gender." *Social Problems* 36 (5): 473–90.

Coney, Sandra. 1994. *The menopause industry: How the medical establishment exploits women.* Alameda, CA: Hunter House.

Connell, Robert. 1987. *Gender and power: Society, the person, and sexual politics.* Stanford, CA: Stanford University Press.

Conrad, Peter. 1985. "The meaning of medications: Another look at compliance." *Social Science and Medicine* 20: 29–37.

————.1987a. "The experience of illness: Recent and new directions." Pp. 1–31 in Julius Roth et al., eds., *The experience and management of chronic illness: Research in the sociology of health care,* Vol. 6. Greenwich, CT: JAI Press.

————. 1987b. "The noncompliant patient in search of autonomy." *Hastings Report* (August): 15–17.

―――. 1992. "Medicalization and social control." *Annual Review of Sociology* 18: 209–32.

Cook, Gareth. 2002. "Man-made womb." *Boston Globe,* March 31, 1.

Cooley, Charles Horton. 1983. *Human nature and the social order.* New Brunswick, NJ: Transaction Publishers.

Coppen, A., and M. Bishop. 1981. "Hysterectomy, hormones and behaviour: A prospective study." *Lancet* 1: 126–28.

Corbin, Juliet, and Anselm L. Strauss. 1985. "Managing chronic illness at home." *Qualitative Sociology* 8: 24–47.

―――. 1987. "Accompaniments of chronic illness: Changes in body, self, biography, and biographical time." Pp. 249–81 in Julius Roth and Peter Conrad, eds., *The experience and management of chronic illness: Research in the sociology of health care,* Vol. 6. Greenwich, CT: JAI Press.

Corea, Gena. 1977. *The hidden malpractice: How American medicine treats women as patients and professionals.* New York: William Morrow.

Cosper, B., S. Fuller, and G. Robinson. 1978. "Characteristics of post-hospitalization recovery following hysterectomy." *Journal of Obstetrical and Gynecological Nursing* 7 (3) (May/June): 7–11.

Costa, Barbara, and D. Dilanni. n.d. *Sudden changes: Post-hysterectomy syndrome.* New York: Cinema Guild. Videocassette.

Cutler, Winnifred B. 1988. *Hysterectomy: Before and after.* New York: Harper and Row.

Cutler, Winnifred Berg, Celso-Ramón Garcia, and David A. Edwards. 1984. *Menopause: A guide for women and the men who love them.* New York: W. W. Norton.

Dally, Ann. (1991). *Women under the knife: A history of surgery.* New York: Routledge.

Daly, Mary. 1978. *Gyn/ecology: The metaethics of radical feminism in the contemporary West.* Berkeley: University of California Press.

Daly, M. J. 1976. "Psychological impact of surgical procedures on women." Pp. 308–13 in H. I. Sadock and A. M. Freedman, eds., *The sexual experience.* Baltimore: Williams and Wilkins.

Darling, Carol Anderson, and Yvonne M. McKoy-Smith. 1993. "Understanding hysterectomies: Sexual satisfaction and quality of life." *Journal of Sex Research* 30 (4) (November): 324–35.

Davis, Fred. 1960. "Uncertainty in medical prognosis: Clinical and functional." *American Journal of Sociology* 66: 41–47.

Deaux, Kay. 1993. "Commentary: Sorry, wrong number—A reply to Gentile's call." In Douglas A. Gentile, Rhoda K. Unger, Mary Crawford, and Kay Deaux, "What is sex anyway?" *Psychological Science* 4 (2): 120–6.

Deaux, Kay, and Mary E. Kite. 1987. "Thinking about gender." Pp. 92–120 in Beth B. Hess and Myra Marx Ferree, eds., *Analyzing Gender*. Newbury Park, CA: Sage.

Deaux, Kay, and Brenda Major. 1990. *A social-psychological model of gender*. New Haven: Yale University Press.

de Beauvoir, Simone. 1989. *The second sex*. New York: Vintage Books.

Delaney, Janice, Mary Jane Lupton, and Emily Toth. 1988. *The curse: A cultural history of menstruation*. New York: Dutton.

Dell, Pippa. 2000. "Deconstructing 'hysterectomized woman': A materio-discursive approach." Pp. 329–39 in Jane M. Ussher, ed., *Women's Health: Contemporary International Perspectives*. Oxford, UK: Blackwell.

Dell, P., and S. Papagiannidou. 1999. "Hysterical talk? A discourse analysis of Greek women's accounts of their experiences following hysterectomy and oophorectomy." *Journal of Reproductive and Infant Psychology* 17 (4): 391–404.

Dennerstein, L., C. Wood, and G. Burrows. 1977a. "Sexual dysfunction following hysterectomy." *Australian Family Physician* 6: 535–43.

———. 1977b. "Sexual response following hysterectomy and oophorectomy." *American Journal of Obstetrics and Gynecology* 49: 92–96.

Derogatis, L. R. 1980. "Breast and gynecologic cancers: Their unique impact on body image and sexual identity in women." *Frontiers in Radiology Therapy and Oncology* 14: 1–11.

Doress-Worters, Paula B., and Diana Laskin Siegal. 1994. *The new ourselves, growing older*. New York: Simon and Schuster.

Dranov, Paula. 1993. *Estrogen: Is it right for you?* New York: Simon and Schuster.

Drelich, Marvin G., and Irving Bieber. 1958. "The psychologic importance of the uterus and its functions." *Journal of Nervous and Mental Diseases* 126 (1) (January): 322–36.

Edelstein, Barbara. 1982. *The woman doctor's medical guide for women: How to look better, feel great, and get the most out of life*. New York: Perigord Press.

Ehrenreich, Barbara, and Deirdre English. 1978. *For her own good: 150 years of the experts' advice to women*. New York: Doubleday.

Elson, Jean.1996. "Castration, hysterectomy, and the construction of 'woman': Medical discourse and women's voices." Paper presented to the Society for the Study of Social Problems, New York.

———. 2000. "'Am I still a woman?': An analysis of gynecological surgery and gender identity." Ph.D. diss., Brandeis University.

———. 2001a. "An analysis of menstruation and gender identity for women who have undergone hysterectomy." Paper presented to the Society for Menstrual Cycle Research, Avon, Conn.

————. 2001b. "'Hormonal hierarchy: Stratification of stigma among women who have experienced hysterectomy." Paper presented to the American Sociological Association, Anaheim, Calif.

————. 2001c. "'Hormonal hierarchy: Stratification of stigma among women who have experienced hysterectomy." Paper presented to the Eastern Sociological Association, Boston.

————. 2002. "Menarche, menstruation, and gender identity: Retrospective accounts from women who have undergone hysterectomy." *Sex Roles* 46 (1/2): 63–81.

————. 2003. "Hormonal hierarchy: Hysterectomy and stratified stigma." *Gender & Society* 17 (5) (October).

Epstein, Cynthia Fuchs. 1988. *Deceptive distinctions*. New Haven, CT: Yale University Press.

Epstein, Steven. 1990. "Gay politics, ethnic identity: The limits of social constructionism." Pp. 239–95 in Edward Stein, ed., *Forms of desire: Sexual orientation and the social constructionist controversy*. New York: Garland.

Erikson, Erik H. 1968. *Identity: Youth and crisis*. New York: W. W. Norton.

Everson, S. A., R. A. Matthews, D. S. Guzick, R. R. Wing, and L. H. Kuller. 1995. "Effects of surgical menopause on psychological characteristics and lipid levels: The healthy woman study." *Health Psychology* (EJL). 14(5) (September): 435–43.

Fageeh, W., H. Raffa, H. Jabbad, A. Marzouki. 2002. "Case report: Transplantation of the human uterus." *International Journal of Gynecology and Obstetrics* (March 7): 245–51.

Farquhar, Cynthia M., and Claudia A. Steiner. 2002. "Hysterectomy rates in the United States 1990–1997." *Obstetrics and Gynecology* 99: 229–34.

Fausto-Sterling, Anne. 1985. *Myths of gender: Biological theories about women and men*. New York: Basic Books.

————. 1987. "Society writes biology/biology constructs gender." *Daedalus* (fall): 61–75.

————. 1993. "The five sexes: Why male and female are not enough." *The Sciences* (March/April): 20–25.

Finley, Christine, Edward W. Gregg, Laura J. Solomon, and Elaine Gay. 2001. "Disparities in hormone replacement therapy use by socioeconomic status in a primary care population." *Journal of Community Health* 26 (1) (February): 39–50.

Firestone, Shulamith. 1970. *The dialectic of sex: The case for feminist revolution*. New York: Morrow.

Fisher, Sue Carole. 1986. *In the patient's best interest: Women and the politics of medical decisions*. New Brunswick, NJ: Rutgers University Press.

Fitzpatrick, Ray, John Hinton, Stanton Newman, Graham Scambler, and James Thompson, eds., 1984. *The experience of illness.* New York: Tavistock.

Foucault, Michel. 1980. *Herculine Barbin: Being the recently discovered memoirs of a nineteenth-century French hermaphrodite.* New York: Pantheon Books.

Fox, Renée. 1957. "Training for uncertainty." Pp. 207–41 in R. K. Merton, G. Reader, and P. L. Kendall, eds., *The student physician.* Cambridge, MA.: Harvard University Press.

Franklin, Pamela. 1991. "Too many hysterectomies." *New Directions for Women* 20 (May/June): 8.

Freidson, Elliot. 1970. *Profession of medicine.* New York: Dodd, Mead.

Fried, Barbara. 1977. "Boys will be boys will be boys: The language of sex and gender." Pp. 37–59 in Ruth Hubbard, Mary Sue Henifen, and Barbara Fried, eds., *Women look at biology looking at women: A collection of feminist critiques.* Boston: G. K. Hall.

Friedan, Betty. 1963. *The feminine mystique.* New York: Norton.

Frye, Marilyn. 1983. *The politics of reality: Essays in feminist theory.* Trumansburg, NY: Crossing Press.

Fugh-Berman, Adriane. 1998. "Phytoestrogens: A new alternative for women?" *Network News,* May/June: 1, 4, 7.

———. 1994. "Man to man at Georgetown: Tales out of medical school." Pp. 47–53 in Karen M. Hicks, ed., *Misdiagnosis: Woman as a disease.* Allentown, PA: People's Medical Society.

Fuss, Diana. 1989. *Essentially speaking.* New York and London: Routledge.

Galler, R. 1984. "The myth of the perfect body." Pp. 165–72 in Carol Vance, ed., *Pleasure and danger.* Boston: Routledge and Kegan Paul.

Galvotti, Christine, and Donna L. Richter. 2000. "Talking about hysterectomy: The experiences of women from four cultural groups." *Journal of Women's Health and Gender-Based Medicine* 9 (Suppl. 2): S-63–S-67.

Galyer, K. T., H. M. Conaglen, A. Hare, and J. V. Conaglen. 1999. "The effect of gynecological surgery on sexual desire." *Journal of Sex and Marital Therapy* 25 (2) (April-June): 81–88.

Garfinkel, Harold. 1967. "Passing and the managed achievement of sex status in an intersexed person." Pp. 116–85 in Harold Garfinkel (ed.), *Studies in ethnomethodology.* Englewood Cliffs, NJ: Prentice-Hall.

Gath, D., P. Cooper, and A. Day. 1982. "Hysterectomy and psychiatric disorder: Levels of psychiatric morbidity before and after hysterectomy." *British Journal of Psychiatry* 140: 335–50.

Gath, D., N. Rose, A. Bond, A. Day, A. Garrod, and S. Hodges. 1995. "Hysterectomy and psychiatric disorder: Are the levels of psychiatric morbidity falling?" *Psychological Medicine* 25(2) (March): 277–83.

Gentry, Carol. 1999. "Sexual activity isn't diminished by hysterectomy, study finds." *Wall Street Journal,* 24 November, B5.

Gilligan, Carol. 1982. *In a different voice: Psychological theory and women's development.* Cambridge, MA: Harvard University Press.

Glaser, Barney G., and Anselm Strauss. 1967. *The discovery of grounded theory.* Chicago: Aldine.

Goffman, Erving. 1959. *The presentation of self in everyday life.* New York: Doubleday.

———. 1963. *Stigma.* Englewood Cliffs, NJ: Prentice Hall.

———. 1976. "Gender display." *Studies in the Anthropology of Visual Communication* 3: 69–77.

———. 1977. "The arrangement between the sexes." *Theory and Society* 4: 301–33.

Goldfarb, Herbert A. 1990. *The no-hysterectomy option: Your body—your choice.* New York: John Wiley.

Golub, Sharon, ed. 1983. *Menarche: The transition from girl to woman.* Lexington, MA: D.C. Heath.

Gonyea, Judith G. 1996. "Finished at fifty: The politics of the menopause and hormone replacement therapy." *American Journal of Preventive Medicine* 12 (5) (September–October): 415–19.

Grady, Denise. 2002a. "Scientists question hormone therapies for menopause ills." *New York Times* (April 18): A1, A20.

———. 2002b. "Medical first: A transplant of a uterus?" *New York Times,* 7 March, sec. A, p. 1, col. 1.

Grady, Deborah, D. Herrington, and V. Bittner et al. for the HERS Research Group. 2002. "Cardiovascular disease outcomes during 6.8 years of hormone therapy: Heart and estrogen/progestin replacement study follow-up (HERS II)." *Journal of the American Medical Society* 288: 49–57.

Gramling, R., and C. J. Forsythe. 1987. "Exploiting stigma." *Sociological Forum* 2:401–15.

Greenhill, J. P. 1954. *Office gynecology,* 6th ed. (Quoted in Lander 1988, *Images of bleeding,* New York: Orlando Press, 65).

Greenwood, Sadja. 1996. *Menopause naturally: Preparing for the second half of life.* Volcano Press.

Greer, Germaine. 1970. *The female eunuch.* New York: Bantam Books.

———. 1992. *The change: Women, aging and the menopause.* New York: Alfred A. Knopf.

Greil, Arthur L. 1991a. "A secret stigma: The analogy between infertility and chronic illness and disability." *Advances in Medical Sociology* 2: 17–38.

———. 1991b. *Not yet pregnant: Infertile couples in contemporary America.* New Brunswick, NJ: Rutgers University Press.

Groff, J., P. D. Mullen, T. Byrd, A. J. Shelton, E. Lees, and J. Goode. 2000. "Decision making, beliefs, and attitudes toward hysterectomy: A focus group study with medically underserved women in Texas." *Journal of Women's Health and Gender-Based Medicine.* 9 (Suppl. 2): S-39–S-50.

Grossman, Marilyn, and Pauline Bart. 1979. "Taking men out of menopause." Pp. 163–84 in Ruth Hubbard, Mary Sue Henfin, and Barbara Fried, eds., *Women looking at biology looking at women.* Boston: G. K. Hall.

Grosz, Elizabeth. 1994. "Sexual difference and the problem of essentialism." Pp. 82–98 in Naomi Schor and Elizabeth Weed, eds., *The essential difference.* Bloomington: Indiana University Press.

Gubrium, Jaber, F. James A. Holstein, and David R. Buckholdt. 1994. *Constructing the life course.* Dix Hills, NY: General Hall.

Guzick, David S., and Kathleen Hoeger. 2000. "Sex, hormones, and hysterectomies." *New England Journal of Medicine* 343 (10) (September 7): 730–31.

Hampton, Peter, and William G. Tarnasky. 1974. "Hysterectomy and tubal ligation: A comparison of the psychological aftermath." *American Journal of Obstetrics and Gynecology* 119 (7) (August 1): 949–52.

Harding, Jennifer. 1998. *Sex acts: Practices of femininity and masculinity.* Thousand Oaks, CA: Sage.

———. 1997. "Bodies at risk: Sex, surveillance and hormone replacement therapy." Pp. 134–50 in Alan Petersen and Robin Bunton, eds., *Foucault, health and medicine.* London: Routledge.

Harris, Dena E., and Helene MacLean. 1992. *Recovering from hysterectomy.* New York: Harper.

Harris, W. J. 1997. "Complications of hysterectomy." *Clinical Obstetrics and Gynecology* 40(4) (December): 939–46.

Hasson, H. M. 1993. "Cervical removal at hysterectomy for benign disease: Risks and benefits." *Journal of Reproductive Medicine* 38 (10) (October): 781–90.

Hawkinson, William Paul. 1959. "Sociological aspects of hysterectomy." Ph.D. diss., Ohio State University.

Helstrom, L., E. Weiner, D. Sorbom, and T. Backstrom. 1994. "Predictive value of psychiatric history, genital pain, and menstrual symptoms for sexuality after hysterectomy." *Acta Obstetrics and Gynecology Scandinavia* 73: 575–80.

Hemminki, E., D. J. Brambilla, S. M. McKinlay, and J. G. Posner. 1991. "Use of estrogens among middle-aged Massachusetts women." *Drug Intelligence and Clinical Pharmacy* 25: 418–23.

Hendricks-Matthews, M. K. 1991. "The importance of assessing a woman's history of sexual abuse before hysterectomy." *Journal of Family Practice* 32 (6): 631–32.

Holmes, Helen Bequaert, and Laura M. Purdy, eds. 1992. *Feminist Perspectives in Medical Ethics*. Bloomington: Indiana University Press.

Houppert, Karen. 1999. *The curse: Confronting the last unmentionable taboo: Menstruation*. New York: Farrar, Straus and Giroux.

Howard, Judith A., and Jocelyn Hollander. 1997. *Gendered situations, gendered selves: A gender lens on social psychology*. Walnut Creek, CA: Altamira Press.

Hrdy, Sarah Blaffer. 1999. *Mother nature: A history of mothers, infants, and natural selection*. New York: Pantheon.

Hubbard, Ruth, Mary Sue Henifen, and Barbara Fried, eds. 1977. *Women look at biology looking at women: A collection of feminist critiques*. Boston: G. K. Hall.

Huffman, J. W. 1985. "Sex after hysterectomy." *Medical Aspects of Human Sexuality* 19: 171–79.

Hufnagel, Vicki. 1989. *No more hysterectomies*. New York: New American Library.

Jackson, Beryl. 1992. "Black women's responses to menarche and menopause." Pp. 178–90 in Alice J. Dan and Linda L. Lewis (eds.), *Menstrual health in women's lives*. Urbana: University of Illinois Press.

Jacobowitz, Ruth S. 1993. *150 Most-asked questions about menopause*. New York: Hearst Books.

Jenkins, Ron. 1998. "Oklahoma senate OKs castration bill." [America On-Line news service]. New York: Associated Press: accessed 3 March.

Johannes, Catherine B., Sybil L. Crawford, Jennifer G. Posner, and Sonja M. McKinlay. 1994. "Longitudinal patterns and correlates of hormone replacement therapy use in middle-aged women." *American Journal of Epidemiology* 140: 439–52.

Jordan, Sandra H. 2002. "An inquiry into women's experience of sexual desire following hysterectomy." Ph.D. diss., Union Institute.

Kaiser, R., M. Kusche, and H. Wurz. 1989. "Hormone levels in women after hysterectomy." *Archives of Gynecology and Obstetrics* 244: 169–73.

Kaltreider, N., A. Wallace, and M. Horowitz. 1979. "A field study of the stress response syndrome: Young women after hysterectomy." *Journal of the American Medical Association* 242 (14): 1499–503.

Karp, David. 1999. "Illness and identity." Pp. 83–93 in Kathy Charmaz and Debora A. Paterniti, eds., *Health, illness, and healing: Society, social context and self: An anthology.* Los Angeles: Roxbury.

Katz, Phyllis A. 1979. "Development of female identity." *Sex Roles* 5 (2) (April): 155–78.

Kaufert, Patricia A. 1982. "Myth and the menopause." *Sociology of Health and Illness* 4 (2) (July): 141–66.

Kaufert, Patricia A., and Sonja M. McKinlay. 1985. "Estrogen replacement therapy: The production of medical knowledge and the emergence of policy." Pp. 113–38 in Ellen Lewin and Virginia Olesen, eds., *Women, health, and healing: Toward a new perspective.* New York and London: Tavistock Publications.

Kaunitz, Andrew M. 2002. "Use of combination hormone replacement therapy in light of recent data from the women's health initiative." *Medscape Women's Health eJournal* (July 12) (http://www.medscape.com).

Kav-Venaki, S., and L. Zakham. 1983. "Psychological effects of hysterectomy in premenopausal Women." *Journal of Psychosomatic Obstetrics and Gynecology* 2: 76–80.

Keith, C. "Discussion group for posthysterectomy patients." *Health and Social Work* 5 (1): 59–63.

Kelley, Kathy. 2001. *Through the Land of Hyster: The Hyster sisters guide.* Denton, TX: Hyster Sisters.

———. 2002. Hystersisters Web site (June) (http://www.hystersisters.com).

Kessler, Susan J., and Wendy McKenna. 1978. *Gender: An ethnomethodological approach.* New York: John Wiley.

Kilkku, P. 1983. "Supravaginal uterine amputation vs. hysterectomy: Effects on coital frequency and dyspareunia." *Acta Obstetrics Gynecological Scandanavia* 62: 141–45.

Kilkku, P., and M. Gronroos. 1982. "Preoperative electrocoagulation of endocervical mucosa and later carcinoma of the cervical stump." *Acta Obstetrics Gynecological Scandanavia* 61: 265–67.

Kilkku, P., M. Gronroos, T. Hirvonen, and L. Rauramo. 1983. "Supravaginal uterine amputation vs. hysterectomy: Effects on libido and orgasm." *Acta Obstetrics Gynecological Scandanavia* 62: 147–52.

Kimball, Meredith. 1995. *Feminist visions of gender similarities and differences.* New York and London: Haworth Press.

Kinnick, Virginia Gramzow, and Debra Woodard Leners. 1995. "The hysterectomy experience: An ethnographic study." *Journal of Holistic Nursing* 13 (2) (June): 142–54.

Kjerulff, K., P. Langenberg, G. Guzinkis. 1993. "The socioeconomic correlates of hysterectomies in the United States." *American Journal of Public Health* 83: 106.

Klein, Renate, and Lynette J. Dumble. 1994. "Disempowering midlife women: The science and politics of hormone replacement therapy (HRT)." *Women's Studies International Forum* 17 (4) (July-August): 327–43.

Koeske, Randi D. 1982. "Toward a biosocial paradigm for menopause research: Lessons and contributions from the behavioral sciences," in A. Voda, M. Dinnerstein, and S. O'Donnell, eds., *Changing perspectives on menopause*. Austin: University of Texas Press.

Koff, Elissa, Jill Rierdan, and S. Jacobsen.1981. "The personal and interpersonal significance of menarche." *Journal of the American Academy of Child Psychiatry* 20: 148–58.

Kolata, Gina. 2002. "Study is halted over rise seen in cancer risk." *New York Times,* July 9, A-1, A-18.

Komesaroff, Paul A., Philipa Rothfield, and Jeanne Daly, eds. 1997. *Reinterpreting menopause: Cultural and philosophical issues.* New York and London: Routledge.

Korenbrot, C., A. B. Flood, M. Higgens et al. 1981. "Case Study #15: Elective Hysterectomy: Costs, Risks, and Benefits." In *The implications of cost-effective analysis of medical technology, background paper #2: Case studies of medical technologies.* Congress of the United States, Office of Technological Assessment (October): 9.

Krull, Julie Kaye. 2000. "A phenomenological investigation of surgically induced menopause." Ph.D. diss., Walden University.

Lalinec-Michaud, M., and F. Engelsmann. 1984. "Depression and hysterectomy: A prospective study." *Psychosomatics* 25: 550–58.

Lalos, A. and O. Lalos. 1996. The partner's view about hysterectomy. *Journal of Psychosomatic Obstetrics and Gynecology* 19 (2): 119–24.

Lander, Louise. 1988. *Images of bleeding: Menstruation as ideology.* New York: Orlando Press.

Laqueur, Thomas. 1990. *Making sex: Body and gender from the Greeks to Freud.* Cambridge, MA: Harvard University Press.

Lark, Susan. 1995. *The estrogen decision self-help book.* Berkeley, CA: Celestial Arts Publishing.

Laurence, Leslie, and Beth Weinhouse. 1994. *Outrageous practices: The alarming truth about how medicine mistreats women.* New York: Fawcett Columbine.

Lee, Janet. 1994. "Menarche and the (hetero)sexualization of the female body." *Gender and Society* 8 (3): 343–62.

———. 1998. "Menarche and the (hetero)sexualization of the female body." Pp. 82–99 in Rose Weitz, ed., *The politics of women's bodies: Sexuality, appearance, and behavior.* New York: Oxford University Press.

Lee, Janet, and Jennifer Sasser-Coen. 1996. *Blood stories: Menarche and the politics of the female body in contemporary U.S. society.* New York: Routledge.

Lees, E., A. J. Shelton, and J. Y. Groff. 2001. "Beliefs and attitudes of middle-aged lesbians about hysterectomy." *Journal of the Gay and Lesbian Medical Association* 5 (1) (March): 3–10.

LeGuin, Ursula. 1976. "The space crone." Pp. 3–6 in *Dancing at the Edge of the World.* New York City: Grove Press.

Lenfant, Claude. 2002. "Dear WHI participant (in the estrogen alone trial)." (July 16) (http://www.whi.org)

Lennon, Mary Clare. 1982. "The psychological consequences of menopause: The importance of timing of a life stage event." *Journal of Health and Social Behavior* 23 (4) (December): 353–66.

Lepine, L. A., S. D. Hillis, P. A. Marchbanks, L. M. Koonin, B. Morrow, B. A. Kieke, et al. 1997. "Hysterectomy surveillance—United States, 1980–1993." Atlanta: *MMWR, National Center for Chronic Disease Prevention and Health Promotion, Centers for Disease Control and Prevention* 46 (SS-4) (August 8): 1–15.

Lewis, Jane. 1993. "Feminism, the menopause and hormone replacement therapy." *Feminist Review* 43 (spring): 38–56.

Linde, V. J., and A. E. Boilesen. 1997. "Hysterectomy and sexual function: A historical view." *Nordisk Sexologi* 15 (2) (August): 109–15.

Lippert, Joan. 1993. "Unnecessary hysterectomies." *Ladies Home Journal* (May): 122.

Lock, Margaret. 1993. *Encounters with aging: Mythologies of menopause in Japan and North America.* Berkeley: University of California Press.

Loft, A., O. Lindegaard, and A. Tabor. 1997. "Incidence of ovarian cancer after hysterectomy: A nationwide controlled follow up." *British Journal of Obstetrics and Gynaecology* 104 (November): 1296–301.

Lorber, Judith. 2000. "Gender hierarchies in the health professions." Pp. 436–45 in Dana Vannoy, ed., *Gender mosaics: Social perspectives: Original readings.* Los Angeles: Roxbury.

———. 1994. *Paradoxes of gender.* New Haven: Yale University Press.

Lorber, Judith, Rose Laub Coser, Alice Rossi, and Nancy Chodorow. 1981. "On *The Reproduction of Mothering*: A methodological debate." *Signs* 6 (3) (spring): 482–500.

Love, Susan (with Karen Lindsey). 1998. *Dr. Susan Love's hormone book: Making informed choices about menopause.* New York: Times Books.

Lupton, Deborah. 1994. *Medicine as culture: Illness, disease and the body in Western societies.* Thousand Oaks, CA: Sage.

Lyons, Antonia C., and Christine Griffin. 2000. "Representations of menopause and women at midlife." Pp. 470–76 in Jane M. Ussher, ed., *Women's health: Contemporary international perspectives.* Oxford, UK: Blackwell.

MacKinnon, Catherine. 1987. *Feminism unmodified.* Cambridge, MA: Harvard University Press.

Marshall, Helen. 1996. "Our bodies ourselves: Why we should add old-fashioned empirical phenomenology to the new theories of the body." *Women's Studies International Forum* 19: 253–65.

Martin, Emily. 1992 [1987]. *The woman in the body: A cultural analysis of reproduction.* Boston: Beacon Press.

Martin, R., W. Roberts, and P. Clayton. 1980. "Psychiatric status after hysterectomy." *Journal of the American Medical Association* 244 (4): 350–53.

Massachusetts Breast Cancer Coalition. 1996. "Genetic testing for heritable breast cancer: What you need to know before considering it." *Stop the Epidemic: The Newsletter of the Massachusetts Breast Cancer Coalition* 9 (Winter): 1, 3.

Matthews, Ralph, and Anne Martin Matthews. 1986. "Infertility and involuntary childlessness: The transition to nonparenthood." *Journal of Marriage and the Family* 48: 641–49.

McClintock, Martha. 1971. "Menstrual synchrony and suppression." *Nature* 229: 244.

McCrea, Frances B. 1983. "The politics of menopause: The 'discovery' of a deficiency disease." *Social Problems* 31 (1) (October): 111–23.

McKinlay, J., S. McKinlay, and D. Brambilla. 1987. "The relative contributions of endocrine changes and social circumstances to depression in mid-aged women." *Journal of Health and Social Behavior* 28: 345–63.

Mead, George Herbert. 1962. *Mind, self, and society: From the standpoint of a social behaviorist,* ed. Charles W. Morris. Chicago: University of Chicago Press.

Mechanic, David. 1968. *Medical sociology.* New York: Free Press.

Meikle, Stuart, H. Brody, and F. Pysh. 1977. "An investigation into the psychological effects of hysterectomy." *Journal of Nervous Mental Disease* 164: 36–41.

Meilahn, E. N., K. A. Matthews, G. Egeland, and S. F. Kelsey. 1989. "Characteristics of women with hysterectomy." *Maturitas* 11: 319.

Melody, George F. 1962. "Depressive reactions following hysterectomy." *American Journal of Obstetrics and Gynecology* 83 (3) (February 1): 410–13.

Mendelsohn, Robert S. 1981. *Male practice: How doctors manipulate women.* Chicago: Contemporary Books.

Meyer, Morris. 1991. "I dream of Jeannie: Transsexual striptease as scientific display." *Drama Review* (spring): 35.

Miall, Charlene E. 1986. "The stigma of involuntary childlessness." *Social Problems* 33: 268–82.

———. 1994. "Community constructs of involuntary childlessness: Sympathy, stigma, and social support." *Canadian Review of Sociology and Anthropology* 31 (4): 392–421.

Miller, P. Y., and M. R. Fowlkes. 1980. "Social and behavioral constructions of female sexuality." *Signs* 5 (Summer): 783–800.

Millet, Kate. 1970. *Sexual politics*. Garden City, NY: Doubleday.

Mingo, Clo, Clara J. Herman, and Maria Jasperse. 2002. "Women's stories: Ethnic variations in women's attitudes and experiences of menopause, hysterectomy, and hormone replacement therapy." *Journal of Women's Health and Gender-based Medicine* 9 (2): S-27–S-38.

Mitchell, Juliet. 1973. *Woman's estate*. New York: Vintage Books.

Money, John, and Anke Ehrhardt. 1972. *Man and woman, boy and girl: The differentiation and dimorphism of gender identity from conception to maturity*. Baltimore: Johns Hopkins University Press.

Montreal Health Press. 1997. *Menopause handbook*. Montreal: Montreal Health Press.

Moore, J. T., and D. M. Tolley. 1976. "Depression following hysterectomy." *Psychosomatics* 17:86–89.

Morgan, Susanne. 1982. *Coping with a hysterectomy: Your own choice, your own solutions*. New York: Dial.

Mosucci, Ornella. 1990. *The science of woman: Gynaecology and gender in England, 1800–1929*. New York: Cambridge University Press.

Murphy, Robert F. 1999. "The damaged self." Pp. 62–71 in Kathy Charmaz and Debora A. Paterniti, eds., *Health, illness, and healing: Society, social context and self: An anthology*. Los Angeles: Roxbury.

Murray, Michael, and Kerry Chamberlain. 2000. "Qualitative methods and women's health research." Pp. 40–50 in Jane Ussher (ed.), *Women's Health: Contemporary International Perspectives*. Oxford, UK: Blackwell.

Nadelson, C. C., M. T. Notman, and E. A. Ellis. 1983. "Psychosomatic aspects of obstetrics and gynecology." *Psychosomatics* 24 (10): 871–84.

Nathorst-Boos, J., B. von Schoultz, and R. Carlstrom. 1993. "Elective ovarian removal and estrogen replacement therapy: Effects on sexual life, psychological well-being, and androgen status." *Journal of Psychosomatic Obstetrics and Gynaecology* 14 (4) (December): 283–93.

National Center for Health Statistics. 1996. Hyattsville, MD: Centers for Disease Control and Prevention.

National Women's Health Network (NWHN). 2002. *The truth about hormone replacement therapy: How to break free from the medical myths of menopause*. Roseville, CA: Prima Publishing.

————. 2001. "Women's health snapshots." *Network News* (May/June): 8.

————. 1995. *Taking hormones and women's health: Choices, risks and benefits.* Washington, DC: NWHN.

Newman, G., and L. E. Newman. 1985. "Coping with the stress of hysterectomy." *Journal of Sex Education and Therapy* 11 (2): 65–68.

Newton, Niles, and Enid Baron. 1976. "Reactions to hysterectomy: Fact or fiction." *Primary Care* 3 (4) (December): 781–801.

Nicholson, Linda. 1994. "Interpreting gender." *Signs: Journal of Women in Culture and Society* 20: 79–105.

Northrup, Christiane. 1998. *Women's bodies, women's wisdom: Creating physical and emotional health and healing.* New York: Bantam Doubleday Dell.

Notman, Malkah T. 1993. "Varieties of menopausal experience: Case histories." Pp. 239–54 in Ruth Formanek, ed., *The meanings of menopause: Historical medical and clinical perspectives.* Hillsdale, NJ: Analytic Press.

Oakley, Anne. 1998. "Science, gender, and women's liberation: An argument against postmodernism." *Women's Studies International Forum* 21 (2) (March-April): 133–46.

Ojeda, Linda. 1992. *Menopause without medicine.* Alameda, CA: Hunter House.

Olesen, Virginia, Leonard Schatzman, Nellie Droes, Diane Hatton, and Nan Chico. 1990. "The mundane ailment and the physical self: Analysis of the social psychology of health and illness." *Social Science and Medicine* 30 (4): 449–55.

Ostriker, Alicia Suskin. 1986. *Stealing the language: The emergence of women's poetry in America.* Boston: Beacon Press.

Oudshoorn, Nellie. 1994. *Beyond the natural body: An archaeology of sex hormones.* London: Routledge.

Palmer, Deanette Lynn. 1984. "The effects of preoperative education, attitude toward having children and sex-role socialization on post-hysterectomy depression and self-esteem in young women." Ph.D. diss., Washington State University.

Parazzini, F., E. Negri, C. La Vecchia, L. Luchini, and R. Mezzopane. 1993. "Hysterectomy, oophorectomy, and subsequent ovarian cancer risk." *Obstetrics and Gynecology* 81 (3) (March): 363–66.

Parker, M., J. Bosscher, D. Barnhill, and R. Park. 1993. "Ovarian management during radical hysterectomy in the premenopausal patient." *Obstetrics and Gynecology* 82 (2) (August): 187–90.

Parsons, Talcott. 1951. *The social system.* Glencoe, IL: Free Press.

Patterson, Ralph M., and James B. Craig. 1963. "Misconceptions concerning the psychological effects of hysterectomy." *American Journal of Obstetrics and Gynecology* 85 (1) (January 1): 104.

Payer, Lynn. 1987. *How to avoid a hysterectomy: An indispensable guide to exploring all your options—before you consent to a hysterectomy.* New York: Pantheon Books.

Petras, Kathryn. 1999. *The premature menopause book.* New York: Avon Books.

Peyrot, Mark, James F. McMurry, and Richard Hedges. 1987. "Living with diabetes: The role of personal and professional knowledge in symptom and regimen management." Pp. 107–46 in Peter Conrad and Julius A. Roth, eds., *Research in the Sociology of Health Care* 6. Greenwich, CT: JAI Press.

Plichta, S. B., and C. Abraham. 1996. "Violence and gynecologic health in women <50 years old." *American Journal of Obstetrics and Gynecology* 174 (3): 903–7.

Plourde, Elizabeth. 1998. *The ultimate rape: What every woman should know about hysterectomies and ovarian removal.* Irvine, CA: New Voice Publications.

Polivy, Janet. 1974. "Psychological reactions to hysterectomy: A critical review." *American Journal of Obstetrics and Gynecology* 118 (3) (February): 417–26.

Puretz, Susan L., and Adelaide Haas. 1993. "Sexual desire and responsiveness following hysterectomy and menopause." *Journal of Women and Aging* 5 (2): 3–15.

Raphael, Beverley. 1978. "Psychiatric aspects of hysterectomy." In J. G. Howells, ed., *Modern Perspectives in the Psychiatric Aspects of Surgery.* London: Macmillan.

Reinharz, Shulamit. 1987. "The social psychology of a miscarriage: An application of symbolic interaction theory and method." Pp. 229–49 in M. J. Deegan and M. Hill, eds., *Women and symbolic interaction.* New York: Allen and Unwin.

———. 1988. "Controlling women's lives: A cross-cultural interpretation of miscarriage accounts." *Research in the Sociology of Health Care* 7: 3–37.

———. 1992. *Feminist methods in social research.* New York: Oxford University Press.

Reinisch, J. M. 1990. *The Kinsey Institute new report on sex.* New York: St. Martin's Press.

Rhodes, Julia C., Kristen H. Kjerulff, Patricia W. Langenberg, and Gay M. Guzinski. 1999. "Hysterectomy and sexual functioning." *Journal of the American Medical Association* 282 (20): 1934–41.

———. 2000. "'Sexual function after hysterectomy': Reply." *Journal of the American Medical Association* 283 (17) (May): 2239.

Rich, Adrienne. 1986a. *Of woman born: Motherhood as experience and institution.* New York: W. W. Norton.

————. 1986b. "Notes toward a political location." Pp. 210–231 in *Blood, bread, and poetry: Selected prose 1979–1985*. New York: W. W. Norton.

Richards, Bruce C. 1978. "Hysterectomy: From women to women." *American Journal of Obstetrics and gynecology* 131 (4) (June 15): 446–52.

Richards, D. H. 1973. "Depression after hysterectomy." *The Lancet* (October): 918–19.

————. 1974. "A post-hysterectomy syndrome." *The Lancet* (October): 983–85.

Richter, Donna L., and Christine Galavotti. 2000. "The role of qualitative research in a national project on decision making about hysterectomy and the use of hormone replacement therapy." *Journal of Women's Health and Gender-based Medicine* 9 (2): S-1–S-3.

Richter, D. L., R. E. McKeown, S. J.Corwin, C. Rheaume, and J. Fraser. 2000. "The role of male partners in women's decision making regarding hysterectomy." *Journal of Women's Health and Gender-based Medicine* 9 (Suppl. 2): S-51–S-61.

Riedel, H., E. Lehmann-Willenbrock, and K. Semm. 1986. "Ovarian failure after hysterectomy." *Journal of Reproductive Medicine* 42 (4): 597–600.

Riessman, Catherine Kohler. 1989. "Women and medicalization: A new perspective." Pp. 190–220 in Phil Brown (ed.), *Perspectives in Medical Sociology*. Belmont, CA: Wadsworth.

————. 1993. *Narrative analysis* (Qualitative research methods, vol. 30). Newbury Park, CA: Sage.

Rock, John A., and John D. Thompson, eds. 1997. *TeLinde's operative gynecology*, 8th ed. Philadelphia and New York: Lippincott-Raven.

Roeske, Nancy C. 1978. "Quality of life factors affecting the response to hysterectomy." *Journal of Family Practice* 7: 483–88.

————. 1979. "Hysterectomy and the quality of a woman's life." *Archives of Internal Medicine* 139: 146–47.

Rogers, Wendy. 1997. "Sources of abjection in western responses to menopause." In Paul A. Komesaroff, Philipa Rothfield, and Jeanne Daly, eds., *Reinterpreting menopause: Cultural and philosophical issues*. New York and London: Routledge.

Roopnarinesingh, S., and T. Gopeesingh. 1982. "Hysterectomy and its psychological aftermath." *West Indian Medical Journal* 31: 131–34.

Rosenberg, Morris. 1981. "The self-concept: Social product and social force." Pp. 593–624 in M. Rosenberg and R. H. Turner, eds., *Social Psychology: Sociological Perspectives*. New York: Basic Books.

Rosenberg, Roslind. 1973. "In search of woman's nature." *Feminist Studies* 3 (Fall)3: 141–54.

Rosenfeld, Nancy, and Dianna W. Bolen. 1999. *Just as much a woman: Your guide to hysterectomy and beyond*. Rocklin, CA: Prima Publishing.

Rosenhand, Vera Ann. 1984. "Menopause and its effect on femininity." Ph.D. diss., School of Psychology, Florida Institute of Technology.

Rossi, Alice, 1977. "Biosocial aspects of parenting." *Daedalus* 106 (Spring): 1–32.

Roth, Julius A. 1963. *Timetables: Structuring the passage of time in hospital treatment and other careers.* Indianapolis: Bobbs-Merrill.

Rozenman, Daniel, and Erick Janssen. 2000. "Sexual function after hysterectomy." *Journal of the American Medical Association* 283 (17) (May): 2238–2239.

Rubin, Rita. 1999. "Increased sexual desire follows hysterectomy." *USA Today,* November 24, D1.

Ruddick, Sarah. 1989. *Maternal thinking.* Boston: Beacon Press.

Russo, N. F. 1976. "The motherhood mandate." *Journal of Social Issues* 32: 143–51.

Ryan, M. L. Dennerstein, and R. Pepperell. 1989. "Psychological aspects of hysterectomy." *British Journal of Psychiatry* 154: 516–22.

Ryan, M. M. 1997. "Hysterectomy: Social and psychosexual aspects." *Baillieres Clinical Obstetrics and Gynecology* 11 (1) (March): 23–36.

Sandelowski, Margarete. 1990. "Fault lines: Infertility and imperiled sisterhood." *Feminist Studies* 16 (1) (spring): 33–51.

Scambler, Graham. 1984. "Perceiving and coping with a stigmatizing condition." Pp. 203–26 in Ray Fitzpatrick, John Hinton, Stanton Newman, Graham Scambler, and James Thompson, eds., *The experience of illness.* New York: Tavistock.

Schneider, Joseph W., and Peter Conrad. 1980. "In the closet with illness: Epilepsy, stigma potential and information control." *Social Problems* 28: 32–44.

———. 1983. *Having epilepsy: The experience and control of illness.* Philadelphia: Temple University Press.

Schneider, Beth E., and Meredith Gould. 1987. "Female sexuality: Looking back into the future." Pp. 120–54 in Beth B. Hess and Myra Marx Ferree, eds., *Analyzing gender: A handbook of social science research.* Newbury Park, CA: Sage.

Schumacher, Dorin. (1990). "Hidden death: The sexual effects of hysterectomy." *Journal of Women and Aging* 2: 49–66.

Schwartz, Lynne Sharon. 1987. "So you're going to have a new body!" Pp. 42–58 in *The melting pot and other subversive stories.* New York: Harper and Row.

Scott, Joan. 1988. *Gender and the politics of history.* New York: Columbia University Press.

Scritchfield, S. A. 1989. "The social construction of infertility: From private matter to social concern." Pp. 99–114 in Joel Best, ed., *Images of issues: Typifying contemporary social problems.* New York City: Aldine de Gruyter.

Scully, D. 1994. *Men who control woman's health: The miseducation of obstetrician-gynecologists.* New York: Teachers College Press.

Segal, Lynne. 2000. "Reclaiming women's sexual agency." Pp. 114–123 in Jane M. Ussher, ed., *Women's Health: Contemporary International Perspectives.* Oxford, UK: Blackwell.

Sexton, Anne.1969. "In celebration of my uterus." *Love Poems.* Boston: Houghton Mifflin.

Shandler, Nina. 1997. *Estrogen the natural way.* New York: Villard Books.

Sheehy, Gail. 1992. *The silent passage.* New York: Random House.

———. 1993. "What smart women ask about menopause." *Ladies Home Journal* (May): 116–19.

Sherwin, B. B., and M. M. Gelfand. 1987. "The role of androgen in the maintenance of sexual functioning in oophorectomized women." *Psychosomatic Medicine* 49: 397–409.

Sherwin, B. B., M. M. Gelfand, and W. Brender. 1985. "Androgen enhances sexual motivation in females: A prospective, crossover study of sex steroid administration in the surgical menopause." *Psychosomatic Medicine* 47: 339.

Shinberg, Diane S. 1998. "An event history analysis of age at last menstrual period: Correlates of natural and surgical menopause among midlife Wisconsin women." *Social Science and Medicine* 46 (10): 1381–96.

Showalter, Elaine. 1987. *The female malady: Women, madness and English culture 1830–1980.* New York: Penguin.

Shumaker, Sally A., Claudine Legault, Leon Thal et al. 2003. "Estrogen plus progestin and the incidence of dementia and mild cognitive impairment in postmenopausal women." *Journal of the American Medical Association* 289: 2651–62.

Shuttle, Penelope, and Peter Redgrove. 1986. *The wise wound: Myths, realities, and meanings of menstruation.* New York: Bantam Books.

Siddle, N., P. Sarrel, and M. Whitehead. 1987. "The effect of hysterectomy on the age at ovarian failure: Identification of a subgroup of women with premature loss of ovarian function and literature review." *Fertility and Sterility* 47 (1) (January): 94–100.

Singer, Eleanor. 1974. "Premature social aging: The social-psychological consequences of a chronic illness." *Social Science and Medicine* 8: 143–51.

Sloan, D. 1978. "The emotional aspects of hysterectomy." *American Journal of Obstetrics and Gynecology* 131 (July 15): 598–605.

Smith, N., and G. Reilly. 1994. "Sexuality and body image: The challenges facing male and female cancer patients." *Canadian Journal of Human Sexuality* 3 (2) (Summer): 145–49.

Smith, Stephen. 2002. "Cost, ethical concern make uterus transplants unlikely in US." *Boston Globe,* March 8.

Smith-Rosenberg, Caroll.1985. *Disorderly conduct: Visions of gender in Victorian America.* New York: A. A. Knopf.

Snitow, Ann. 1990. "A gender diary." Pp. 9–43 in Marianne Hirsch and Evelyn Fox Keller, eds., *Conflicts in feminism.* New York: Routledge.

Snitow, Ann, Christine Stansell, and Sharon Thompson, eds. 1983. *Powers of desire.* New York: Monthly Review Press.

Spelman, Elizabeth. 1988. *Inessential woman: Problems of exclusion in feminist thought.* Boston: Beacon Books.

Squier, Susan. 2000. "Fetishism and hysteria: The economies of feminism ex utero." *Journal of Medical Humanities* 21 (2): 59–69.

Stein, Carol. 1991. "The relationship of hysterectomy surgery and self-perception of femininity to mood and sexual satisfaction." Ph.D. diss., California School of Professional Psychology.

Stensrude, Janice. 1996. "The uterus: A necessary loss?" *A Friend Indeed* 12 (9) (February): 1–3.

Stokes, Naomi Miller. 1986. *The castrated woman: What your doctor won't tell you about hysterectomy.* New York: Franklin Watts.

Stolberg, Sheryl Gay. 1999. "Buying years for women on the biological clock." *New York Times,* October 3, sec. 4, pp. 1, 6.

Stoll, Claric? Stasz. 1974. *Female and male: Socialization, social roles, and social structure.* Dubuque, IA: Wm. C. Brown.

Stoller, Robert J. 1968. *Sex and gender.* Vol. 1, *The development of masculinity and femininity.* New York: Jason Aronson.

Strauss, Anselm. 1959. *Mirrors and masks: The search for identity.* Glencoe, IL: Free Press.

Strauss, Helen May. 1968. "Reference group and social comparison processes among the totally blind." In H. H. Hyman and El Singer, eds., *Readings in Reference Group Theory.* Glencoe, IL: Free Press.

Strauss, Anselm L., Juliet Corbin, Shizuko Fagerhaugh, Barney G. Glaser, David Maines, Barbara Suczek, and Carolyn L. Wiener. 1984. *Chronic illness and the quality of life.* St. : Louis: Mosby.

Strausz, Ivan K. 1993. *You don't need a hysterectomy: New and effective ways of avoiding major surgery.* Reading: Addison-Wesley.

Sumner, William Graham. 1960. *Folkways.* New York: New American Library.

Taylor, Dean, and Amber Coverdale Sumrall. 1991. *Women of the fourteenth moon.* Trumansburg, NY: Crossing Press.

Thomas, W. I., and Dorothy Thomas. 1928. *The child in America: Behavior problems and programs.* New York: Knopf.

Todd, Alexandra Dundas. 1989. *Intimate adversaries: Cultural conflict between doctors and women patients.* Philadelphia: University of Pennsylvania Press.

Travis, Cheryl Brown. 1985. "Medical decision making and elective surgery: The case of hysterectomy." *Risk Analysis* 5: 241–51.

Tuana, Nancy. 1993. "With many voices: Feminism and theoretical pluralism." Pp. 28–90 in Paula England, ed., *Theory on gender/feminism on theory.* New York: Aldine DeGreyter.

Turnbull, Colin M. 1985. "Processional ritual among the Mbuti pygmies." *Drama Review* 29 (fall): 6–17.

Turner, Bryan S. 1992. *Regulating bodies: Essays in medical sociology.* London and New York: Routledge.

Turner, Victor. 1969. "The ritual process." Ithaca, NY: Cornell University Press.

Turpin, T. and D. Heath. 1979. "The link between hysterectomy and depression." *Canadian Journal of Psychiatry* 24: 247–252.

Twain, Shania, and Robert John Lange.1997. "Man! I feel like a woman!" *Come on over.* New York: Mercury Records.

Unger, Rhoda Kessler, and Mary Crawford. 1993. "Commentary: Sex and gender—the troubled relationship between terms and concepts." In Douglas A. Gentile, Rhoda K. Unger, Mary Crawford, and Kay Deaux, "What is sex anyway?" *Psychological Science* 4 (2): 120–26.

Ussher, Jane M. 1989. *The psychology of the female body.* London: Routledge.

———. 1992. "Reproductive rhetoric and the blaming of the body." Pp. 31–61 in P. Nicholson and J. Ussher, eds., *The psychology of women's health and health care.* London: Macmillan.

Utian, Wolf. 1975. "Effect of hysterectomy, oophorectomy and estrogen therapy on libido." *International Journal of Obstetrics and Gynecology* 13: 97–100.

Utian, Wulf H., and Ruth S. Jacobowitz. 1990. *Managing your menopause.* New York: Prentice Hall.

Vines, G. 1993. *Raging hormones: Do they rule our lives?* London: Virago.

Voda, Ann M. 1997. *Menopause, me and you: The sound of women pausing.* Binghamton: Haworth Press.

Wallis, Claudia. 1995. "The estrogen dilemma." *Time,* June 26, 51.

Webb, C., and J. Wilson-Barnett. 1983. "Self-concept, social support and hysterectomy." *International Journal of Nursing Studies* 20 (2): 97–107.

Webber, Tammy.1999. "Hysterectomy can improve sex life." America On-Line news service, 24 November (http://www.aol.com).

Weed, Susan. 1991. *Menopausal years: The wise woman way.* Woodstock, NY: Ash Tree Publishing.

Weinrich, James. 1990. "Reality or social construction?" Pp. 175–209 in Edward Stein, *Forms of desire: Sexual orientation and the social constructionist controversy.* New York: Garland.

Weinstein, Sheryl. 1997. "New attitudes toward menopause." *FDA Consumer* 31 (2).

Weiss, Rick. 1999. "Transplant may delay age limits in giving birth." *Boston Globe,* September 24: A1, A21.

Wendell, Susan. 1996. *The rejected body: Feminist philosophical reflections on disability.* New York: Routledge.

West, Candace, and Don H. Zimmerman. 1987. "Doing gender." *Gender and Society* 1: 125–51.

West, Stanley. 1994. *The hysterectomy hoax: A leading surgeon explains why 90% of all hysterectomies are unnecessary and describes all the treatment options available to every woman, no matter what age.* New York: Doubleday.

Williams, Simon J., and Gillian Bendelow. 1998. *The lived body: Sociological themes, embodied issues.* London and New York: Routledge.

Williams, Wanda Wigfall. 1982. *Hysterectomy: Learning the facts, coping with the feelings, facing the future.* New York: Michael Resend.

Williamson, M. L. 1992. "Sexual adjustment after hysterectomy." *Journal of Obstetrics and Gynecological Neonatal Nursing* 21 (1) (January-February): 42–47.

Wolf, S. R. 1970. "Emotional reactions to hysterectomy." *Postgraduate Medicine* 47 (5): 165–69.

Worcester, Nancy, and Mariamne H. Whatley. 1992. "The selling of HRT: Playing on the fear factor." *Feminist Review* 41 (Summer): 1–26.

Woods, Nancy Fugate. 1986. "Socialization and social context: Influence on perimenstrual symptoms, disability, and menstrual attitudes." Pp. 28–29 in Virginia L. Olesen and Nancy Fugate Woods, eds., *Culture, society, and menstruation.* Washington, DC: Hemisphere Publishing Corporation.

Wukasch, Ruth N. 1996. "The impact of a history of rape and incest on the posthysterectomy experience." *Health Care for Women International* 17 (1) (January-February): 47–55.

Zerubavel, Eviatar. 1981. *Hidden rhythms: Schedules and calendars in social life.* Chicago: University of Chicago Press.

Zimmerman, Mary K. 1987. "The women's health movement: A critique of medical enterprise and the position of women." Pp. 442–73 in Beth B. Hess and Myra Marx Ferree, eds., *Analyzing gender: A handbook of social science research.* Newbury Park, CA: Sage.

Zola, Irving Kenneth. 1972. "Medicine as an institution of social control." *Sociological Review* 20: 487–504.

Zussman, L., S. Zussman, R. Sunley, and E. Bjornson. 1981. "Sexual response after hysterectomy-oophorectomy: Recent studies and reconsideration of psychogenesis." *American Journal of Obstetrics and Gynecology* 140: 725–29.

Index